Migraines FOR DUMMIES®

by Diane Stafford and
Jennifer Shoquist, MD

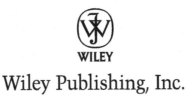

WILEY

Wiley Publishing, Inc.

Migraines For Dummies®

Published by
Wiley Publishing, Inc.
111 River Street
Hoboken, NJ 07030
www.wiley.com

 is a trademark of Wiley Publishing, Inc.

About the Authors

Diane Stafford: The co-author of *Migraines For Dummies*, Diane Stafford knows the subject of migraines personally, having lived with headaches life-long and having grown up in a family of migraine sufferers — sister, brother, and father. Her experiences provided helpful insight on the many challenges that migraineurs face at home, at work, and at play. In this book, she shares numerous ideas for headache management. Diane's main reason for writing this book is the belief that it will help other migraine sufferers lead more fulfilling lives.

Despite migraines, Diane Stafford has been a high-energy writer and magazine editor for twenty-five years. She has served as editor-in-chief of *Houston Health & Fitness Magazine, Dallas-Fort Worth Health & Fitness Magazine, Texas Woman Magazine, Houston Home & Garden, Dallas-Fort Worth Home & Garden, and Philanthropy in Texas.* Also an entrepreneur, Stafford co-owned *Health & Fitness* and helped with startups of the magazine in New Orleans, Philadelphia, and Atlanta. She has written hundreds of articles. She now edits books for Arte Publico Press in Houston and writes books.

Stafford lives with her husband, David Garrett, in Houston, where she is a well-known writer and a community volunteer for Casa de Esperanza de los Ninos and the Emergency Aid Coalition Clothes Center.

Diane Stafford and Jennifer Shoquist (Stafford's daughter) have also co-authored *Potty Training For Dummies* (Wiley Publishing), *No More Panic Attacks: A 30-Day Plan for Conquering Anxiety* (New Page Books), and *The Encyclopedia of Sexually Transmitted Diseases* (to be published by Facts on File, Inc. in 2003).

Jennifer Shoquist, MD: Evaluating and treating patients' headaches is a staple of family practice doctors, and that has also been the case for Dr. Jennifer Shoquist, who teamed up with health writer Diane Stafford to write *Migraines For Dummies* — a book that ambitiously tackles every facet of migraine living, from choosing medications to understanding dietary and exercise triggers to handling people who think your headaches are "in your head."

Jennifer's interest in writing began when she was attending the High School for the Performing and Visual Arts, while also interning at *Health & Fitness Magazine* in Houston, Texas. Later, she completed her medical degree at the University of Texas Medical School at Houston, followed by family practice residency at Memorial Southwest Hospital.

Today, she writes books and serves as a health-issues resource for journalists. She and her husband, Robert San Luis, live in Houston with their son, Benjamin (born during the course of writing this book), and two shih-tzus, Lucy and Sophie.

Dedication

To Allen, Camilla, and Clinton, who never let migraines slow them down. To migraine sufferers everywhere, our fondest wishes that you will find excellent relief from your headache pain. And, finally, we dedicate this book to the newest member of our clan: baby Ben.

Author's Acknowledgments

This great project came our way thanks to the efforts of our incredible literary agent — Elizabeth Frost-Knappman of New England Publishing Associates.

Also, we appreciate the hard work and talent of our wonderful Project Editor, Kathleen Dobie, our capable Acquisitions Editor, Natasha Graf, and our copy editor, Greg Pearson, all at Wiley. We also owe thanks to Dr. Stephen Silberstein, who reviewed the book for technical accuracy. And a special thanks to Houston neurologist Dr. Brian Loftus (loftusmd.com).

Thanks to our wonderful friends and family: David Nordin, Gina and Curtis Bradley, Cameron Liem, Lindsay Liem, Camilla and Richard Pierce, Britt Pierce, Allen and Christina Shirley, Austin Shirley, Xanthe Shirley, Chris Fleming, Dana Chandler, Eddi Lee, Renee Somoza, Rachel Capote, Joanne Goldstein, Dinah Anderson, Donna Pate, Jami Exner.

From Diane: Deep appreciation goes to you, David, for support, friendship, and computer rescues. Loving thanks to my dear daughter Jenny — you've made my life wonderful by being sweet and kind and the love of my life. How fun that you're a terrific co-author, too! And thanks to my son-in-law, Robert, who is always supportive and kind.

From Jennifer: Thank you, Robert, for being so truly great. Thank you, two-month-old Ben, for letting me finish this book. Thank you, Mom, for being the best mom I could imagine (and for being so easy to work with)! I also want to thank Martin and Sarah Shoquist, Dr. Leticia Carlos San Luis, Dr. Tom and Gina Cartwright, Lina Carlos, Wendy Corson, Kristina Holt, Shannon, John, and Jordan Mathis, Christy Waites, Shari Belmarez, my "brother" Austin Shirley, and Sophie and Lucy. To my friends and patients, I send best wishes for migraine-pain-free days.

Publisher's Acknowledgments

We're proud of this book; please send us your comments through our Dummies online registration form located at www.dummies.com/register/.

Some of the people who helped bring this book to market include the following:

Acquisitions, Editorial, and Media Development

Project Editor: Kathleen A. Dobie

Acquisitions Editor: Natasha Graf

Copy Editor: Greg Pearson

Technical Reviewer: Dr. Stephen Silberstein

Editorial Manager: Christine Meloy Beck

Editorial Assistants: Melissa Bennett, Elizabeth Rea

Cover Photos: © Bruce Ayres/Getty Images

Cartoons: Rich Tennant, www.the5thwave.com

Production

Project Coordinator: Kristie Rees

Layout and Graphics: David Batholomew, Amanda Carter, Brian Drumm, Kelly Emkow, Clint Lahnen, Kristin McMullan, Tiffany Muth, Brent Savage, Jeremy Unger

Special Art: Kathryn Born

Proofreaders: John Greenough, Angel Perez, Rob Springer, TECHBOOKS Production Services

Indexer: TECHBOOKS Production Services

Special Help:

Patricia Yuu Pan

Publishing and Editorial for Consumer Dummies

Diane Graves Steele, Vice President and Publisher, Consumer Dummies

Joyce Pepple, Acquisitions Director, Consumer Dummies

Kristin A. Cocks, Product Development Director, Consumer Dummies

Michael Spring, Vice President and Publisher, Travel

Brice Gosnell, Publishing Director, Travel

Suzanne Jannetta, Editorial Director, Travel

Publishing for Technology Dummies

Andy Cummings, Vice President and Publisher, Dummies Technology/General User

Composition Services

Gerry Fahey, Vice President of Production Services

Debbie Stailey, Director of Composition Services

Contents at a Glance

Table of Contents

Introduction

A bout 28 million Americans have migraine headaches. And, if you're one of them, you know all too well that it's hard to predict what a day will hold. Any morning, afternoon, or evening, you may find yourself in the throes of mind-boggling pain, not to mention nausea, vomiting, and sensitivity to loud noises.

So, you've gotten fairly expert at composing migraine metaphors:

> My head's getting pounded by unfriendly fire.

> Contortionists are busting a move in my skull.

Descriptive words just pop out, borne of disbelief that you could actually be hurting so badly.

As a matter of fact, migraines have been driving people nuts forever. Ancient "caregivers" bored holes in people's heads to try to relieve headache pain. Egyptians tied an herb-stuffed clay crocodile to an aching head.

Yet despite a history of being guinea pigs and a yen for spicy metaphors, migraine sufferers remain optimistic. Migraines hurt and can be very disabling, so bring on the remedies!

Knowledge is a powerful weapon in any fight and, in this book, we aim to arm you with the tools you need to whip your migraines into submission.

About This Book

Serving as a reference book for people who want to transition from being hamstrung by headaches to developing high-level pain-busting savvy, *Migraines For Dummies* has parts that are set up as freestanding units. You can peruse each one separately, and feel no urgency about reading chapters or parts in order. After scanning the Table of Contents, zero in on those topics that interest you most, and later, you can turn back to the others.

To tame the migraine beast, you must acknowledge the formidable creature. Denying what you are dealing with does not help. *Migraines For Dummies* provides headache information that helps you understand what you're up against — and a list of remedies effective enough to merit high-roller status in any migraine circle in the world.

Migraines For Dummies offers hope, with a focused, fleshed-out program that works in the real world. Headache medications have their place in the picture, but you absolutely can do more.

The quest for answers — and the pilgrimage to a better health place — is at the core of this book. Essentially, *Migraines for Dummies* will benefit people who want to improve their lives. If you have migraines regularly, you know how devastating they can be. Sometimes, just the thought of making plans seems pointless — what if you get a headache? Friends may think that you're just making excuses to get out of going somewhere. Better not take a chance. So you grow afraid to venture too far from the safety of home base.

In *Migraines For Dummies,* we look at the whole spectrum of the problem, from dealing with the number-one issue of pain relief to handling peripheral problems: absences from work, skepticism from friends, and impact on family. The authors also investigate women's hormonal headaches, stress-as-a-factor in headaches, children's migraines, seniors' head troubles, sex headaches, and sleep-habit demons.

Questions answered

The migraine mob needs health advocates. And we, the authors of *Migraines For Dummies,* fill that role, offering valuable tips on ways to eliminate the fisticuffs going on inside your head in the wacky world of managed health care. *Migraines For Dummies* hands you a gilded invitation to join a proactive group of migraine-busters. Via this book, we provide answers to the following pressing questions:

- How can you know that you have migraines and not some other kind of headache?
- Can your headaches be migraines if you don't have the visual disturbances you've heard are the benchmark sign of a migraine?
- Who's the right doctor for diagnosing and treating your headaches?
- Is there any way to get rid of a migraine once it moves in and sets up camp?
- Do remedies like biofeedback or hypnosis really help the pain?
- How can you find the medication that will provide full-fledged pain relief?
- How can you deal with family and work issues when people really don't understand how debilitating migraines can be?

Truly, because of its complexity, migraine-busting must be considered an extreme sport. You need a concrete headache-management plan, and you need it pronto.

Solutions offered

Check out the many things that *Migraines For Dummies* can do for you:

- ✔ Help you take charge of your headache fate: You don't have to be at the mercy of migraines. You can pave the way to a more headache-free existence. We show you how.

- ✔ Foster a team approach: You can get your mate and children on board, fill in your work supervisor, and cope ably with all of those in your universe whose support can be invaluable during headache episodes.

- ✔ Separate fact from fiction: No, migraines aren't fantasies; they're located in your head, all right, but they're not "all in your head," as some unsympathetic folks may tell you. We sort through the myths and misconceptions.

- ✔ Steer your pain-shedding and migraine-handling: You'll master the technique of warding off a headache, if possible; if not, you'll bash it after it gets going. You'll figure out what to do — and, just as important, what *not* to do.

- ✔ Show you how to stay on message: We get you feeling powerful about conquering migraines and keep you on track by providing answers.

- ✔ Prepare you for all scenarios: From finding out how to function during a migraine haze, to handling health insurance questions, to deciding whether to go to work or school with a headache, we address common problems that migraineurs face.

Caution given

This book contains our opinions and ideas. We intend to provide helpful information on migraines, but we don't offer professional medical, health, or any other kind of personal services via the book.

This is a supplement, not a replacement, for medical advice from your personal healthcare provider. In no way does reading this book replace the need for an evaluation by a physician.

If you want or need personal advice or guidance, please consult a medical, health, or other competent professional — especially if you have a condition that may require medical diagnosis or attention — before adopting any of the suggestions in the book or drawing inferences from the information given.

Foolish Assumptions

Because you picked up this book, we assume a few things about you:

✔ You think that you have migraines, know that you have migraines, or live with, and love, someone with migraines.

You're familiar with the debilitating factor, and you're looking for ideas that will be inspiring, instructive, and winning. You're putting your migraine history and its frustrations behind you. Now you want to venture into the new and promising era of *Migraines For Dummies*. You're saying, "Hit me with your best shot, 'cause I've got nowhere to go but up!"

✔ You may have yet to find a remedy that gets rid of your head pain.

✔ You find the entire migraine problem and its related issues (work, family, public skepticism) somewhat daunting. This idea alone, not to mention the incredible pain, may have inspired you to pick up this book.

✔ You're baffled, unsure of what to do and when to do it — when to take an over-the counter remedy, when to resort to a prescription drug, or whether to try alternative or complementary treatments.

✔ We half-assume that you inherited the migraine tendency, because these headaches run in families.

If you grew up with a parent who had migraines, you're all too familiar with how this 'disability' can alter family plans and dynamics (can you say Bleak House?).

✔ Our biggest assumption is that you're itching to discover ways to get rid of migraine pain, and we think that you can definitely find what you need in this book. We present clear and comprehensive information about all aspects of migraines, along with tips, encouragement, and reassurance.

How This Book Is Organized

This guide to understanding and handling migraines is divided into 7 parts and 26 chapters. You can read the parts randomly — without having to read what came before. If a section requires prior knowledge, we refer you to the chapter number so that you can flip to those pages and get the skinny. Here, we give you a rundown of each part and what's in store for you.

Part I: Looking at the Big Picture: Migraines Demystified

In these chapters, we expose the headaches that perplex and vex you. You get an overview of the things you can do to get rid of them (ideally) or to cope more effectively. We guide you through the maze of reality versus rumor, and we give you a heads-up on the physiology of a headache — and tell you how your family history may have set you up for head pain (in other words, you inherited the migraine proclivity).

We look at recurring headaches that aren't disease-based — as well as at the more ominous sort, characterized by the very important words *new onset* or *worst-ever*. (The latter can sometimes stem from anything from a stroke to a brain hemorrhage to meningitis.)

Also in Part I, we address how to avoid rebound headaches and subdue migraine-associated nausea and vomiting.

You can also take a look at potential headache instigators that can make your head hurt and use the handy headache journal to keep track of your triggers.

Part II: Getting Diagnosed

Part II investigates headaches that sometimes impersonate migraines — cluster and tension-type — and pinpoints the markers of headaches caused by disease.

To reach a conclusion on your headache type (if that's still up in the air), you must enlist a good doctor (Chapter 6), who can evaluate and diagnose your problem or refer you to a headache specialist. You then huddle with your doctor to draw up a battle plan.

We brief you on tests that may be required to determine what's wrong and walk you though designing a treatment plan.

Part III: Giving Migraines a Knockout Punch

Part III ushers you into the "taking care of pain" realm — over-the-counter (OTC) remedies and prescription drugs. This section features a compendium of medications and discusses the good, the bad, and the ugly of each one. We review how abortives work — the meds you take when a migraine's in place — and how prophylactics can be used to stave off trouble.

You can check out complementary and alternative migraine remedies, such as visualization, relaxation techniques, biofeedback, acupuncture, hypnotism, and more. Plus, we tell you how to handle decision-making when you're in a migraine haze and how to negotiate the ER wisely.

Part IV: Committing to Lifestyle Changes

You probably can't live exactly the way you used to and still manage to decrease the number and severity of your migraines — that's the hard, cold fact of it.

The chapters in this part deal with table truths for migraineurs — the do's and don'ts of food and beverage. We list workouts that can help migraine sufferers, and the kinds of movement that tend to spur migraines. We give you tips for checking out your environment for migraine-causing culprits and advice on examining the migraine and sleep-habit link.

Part V: Staying Connected to the People in Your Life

We bring you productive ways to deal with those who think migraine pain is "all in your head." We tell you how to recruit friends and family for your support staff and how to make your mate a staunch ally instead of a grumbler who's tired of hearing "Not tonight, honey — I have a headache."

We give you tips on handling your boss and colleagues — and yourself — in the workplace.

Part VI: Managing Special-Situation Migraines

Part VI cautions you to stay vigilant for signs that big trouble is brewing inside your head. You need to know when the hammering isn't "just a migraine" but a symptom of disease.

Knowing that hormonal swings throw up headache roadblocks for women, we discuss femme migraine details (Chapter 19). Chapter 20 focuses on children's migraines. In the chapter on sex migraines, we separate the serious from the benign (but obnoxious). Chapter 22 examines stress-related migraines, while Chapter 23 talks about seniors and their headaches.

Part VII: The Part of Tens

Here, you get a hodgepodge of good ideas: effective ways to deal compassionately with the migraine-free around you, ways NOT to treat migraines, and terrific tips for support-folks who love migraineurs.

Conventions and Icons Used in This Book

To avoid the "he or she" rigmarole, we solved the pronoun problem by using male pronouns in even-numbered chapters and female pronouns in the odd-numbered chapters.

For Dummies books use snazzy pictures in the margins to draw your attention to specific bits of text. In this book, the pictures we use are

Tack this tidbit on your bulletin board!

Cautions you about practices and procedures you should talk to a doctor about and tells you when you should head for the emergency room.

The dry medical info that you may or may not be interested in is highlighted with this icon. You can skip it if you like.

This icon says: "Here's a valuable morsel you may want to read several times."

This icon alerts you to danger signs and practices to avoid.

Stories about how other migraineurs have coped have this icon beside them.

Where to Go from Here

With the intros tucked away, we usher you into the meat of the book. Look for the parts you need first, and flag others for a look later.

- ✔ If your headaches haven't been diagnosed, start with Parts I and II, which acquaint you with the different types of headaches and give you tips on what your doctor will need from you to make a firm diagnosis.

- ✔ Check out Parts III, IV, and V to find out how to deal with your migraines medically, practically, and socially.

- ✔ If you're a parent, friend, mate, or employer of a migraineur, and you're searching for ways to help and understand, start with Part VII, and then go to Parts III, IV, and V.

As you find parts that help you, flag them for rereading. This book is packed with options, and you have an excellent forecast for getting your headache-future in tow. So let's get started!

Part I

Looking at the Big Picture: Migraines Demystified

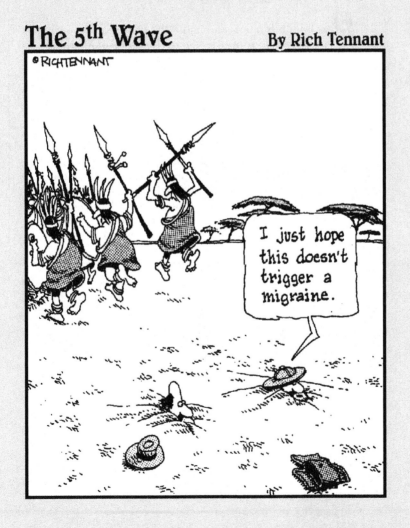

Part

Looking at the Big

Picture: Migraines

Demystified

In this part . . .

*P*art I pitches a tent and lights the campfire, preparing you for an upfront briefing on the Rules of Migraines. You find out quickly that even though these headaches are as common to the populace as s'mores are to summer camp, the wacky things still remain shrouded in mystery. And if you don't understand migraine-criteria, you're left lurking on the fringes of the circle, uncertain whether you belong.

So the job of Part I is to shed some light on migraines for cranial-headache campers, providing a rundown on migraine symptoms, the hereditary factor, and rebound caveats. Having an overview of these dastardly headaches, you stand poised and ready to sing your many merit-badge-worthy migraine-managing achievements.

Chapter 1

Knowing What You're Dealing With: An Overview

About 28 million Americans have migraine headaches. According to the National Headache Foundation's report on the American Migraine Study II, about 53 percent of migraine sufferers have headache pain that causes severe impairment or forces them to retreat to bed. And, the Excedrin Headache Resource Center reports that more than 80 percent of migraineurs have at least some headache-related disability; 50 percent or more, mild or moderate disability (inability to work or do usual activities); and 30 percent, severe disability. By age 15, about 75 percent of children have had a significant headache, and 28 percent of girls 15 to 19 appear to have migraines, according to *Headache and Migraine in Childhood and Adolescence* edited by Vincenzo Guidetti, George Russell, Matti Sillanpaa, and Paul Winner.

Unfortunately, migraines cause children to miss school and adults to miss work. In fact, some employers grow so leery of migraine-ridden employees that they look askance at this kind of problem. To them, it translates to diminished attendance and low productivity. And, according to a study published in *Archives of Internal Medicine* (April 1999), employers have reason for their interpretation: The study cited migraine costs of $13 billion a year for American employers due to employees' missed work and lower productivity.

Getting a Take on What Migraines Are and What They Aren't

Migraines are intense, recurring headaches, but they aren't always debilitating, and they usually are manageable — if you take the time to sort out what kinds of things trigger your migraines, and what sorts of medications and lifestyle changes can make a big difference.

What migraines are

A common myth states that any bad headache, by virtue of being excruciating, must be a migraine. The truth, however, is that some migraines are mild to moderate (although many are severe, indeed). Some other types of headaches — tension, for example — can be extremely painful, too, as can headaches caused by more serious problems such as a hemorrhage (bleeding) in the brain.

The symptoms for migraines may take on many different traits in different people. The uniqueness of the symptoms, in fact, is one reason that some *migraineurs* (people who get migraine headaches) end up living for years without appropriate and effective medication at hand — they don't realize that their headaches are, in fact, migraines.

For example, you may assume, based on what you've heard or what "everyone says," that the headaches you get simply can't be migraines because you don't experience the symptoms that those old wives of "old wives' tale" fame say make a headache a migraine. The truth, however, is that migraines have a wide variety of symptoms, and not every migraine sufferer has the classic symptoms.

Symptoms of migraine headaches include, but are not limited to:

- You feel a throbbing or hammering pain on one or both sides of your head.
- The pain ranges from moderate to severe to almost intolerable.
- You may experience an *aura* (typically, a visual disturbance that lasts from a few minutes to less than an hour, or numbness and tingling of the mouth area and arms), although it's more common that migraine sufferers don't experience auras. Auras usually take place an hour or less before the headache.
- When you have a headache, you may feel lethargic and sad.
- Along with the headache, you may experience nausea, vomiting, malaise, an extreme sensitivity to light, smells, and/or sounds, and periods of no appetite.

Generally speaking, the following are some key features that characterize migraine sufferers:

- ✔ You come from a family that has other migraine-prone family members — your parents, grandparents, or siblings.
- ✔ Your headaches can last from several hours to two or three days.
- ✔ Sleep usually helps you feel better.

Your headache frequency can be several times a week, once a month, or even less often than that. And, migraines can make their presence felt before and after the actual headache. A day or two before your headache, you may experience symptoms such as yawning, frequent urination, drowsiness, irritability, and/or euphoria. After a headache, you may experience a *pain hangover* — you're tired, you don't feel hungry, and your thinking process seems slower.

A migraine is essentially a headache and more. Because your central nervous system's normal state of functioning is disrupted during a migraine, all your body systems are affected. As a result, you may be bothered by sounds, smells, and lights, or your scalp may feel tender, or your feet and hands may be cold.

It's widely agreed that the symptoms of migraines can be different for each individual, so don't assume that your headaches aren't migraines just because you lack auras or other classic symptoms. For example, you may describe your pain as splitting, while the classic symptom is more of a throbbing headache. You may happen to have generalized head pain instead of the classic one-sided misery. Or, you may have never experienced visual disturbances, nausea, or vomiting. Most migraineurs do experience light sensitivity, but maybe you never have. So tell your doctor about your symptoms, and let her be the one to identify the kind of headaches you're suffering from and determine what can be done to wipe out the pain.

In many people, migraines occur because they have a genetic tendency to get headaches — a body-system glitch leads to neurochemical changes that spiral, resulting in chemical shenanigans that affect blood vessels, altering blood flow to your brain and causing your head to ache. (See Chapter 3.)

What migraines aren't

The other main types of headaches have symptoms that are different from those of migraines — but sometimes symptoms overlap, making diagnosis difficult. (See Chapter 4 for information on headaches often confused with migraines.)

Some signs that your headache *isn't* a migraine:

- ✔ Your head pain can best be described as a dull ache.
- ✔ Your shoulder and neck muscles feel knotted-up.
- ✔ You have headaches only after sex or physical exertion.
- ✔ Your headaches are getting steadily worse.

Tripping through the Types of Headaches

Consider the following indicators of these common headache types:

- ✔ **Migraines:** The key symptoms that most healthcare providers look for are a throbbing head pain that's typically one-sided, intensity that's moderate to severe, and a lengthy duration (migraines can range from a few hours up to several days). Activity may make you feel even worse. You may have accompanying nausea and vomiting, and/or sensitivity to light and sound. If you suffer from migraines, you usually have headaches on a regular basis.

- ✔ **Tension-type headaches:** With this type of headache, you have a dull ache characterized by mild to moderate pain. The aching is on both sides of your head, and it comes on slowly.

  If you feel pain around your neck and the back of your head, or in the forehead and temple region — and if the pain feels more like tightness than it does a throbbing or pounding — then you probably have a tension-type headache. You won't have nausea or auras with this kind of headache. Tension-type headaches can occur very frequently (even daily) and are sometimes very painful.

- ✔ **Cluster headaches:** This headache is characterized by sudden and severe piercing pain on one side of the head. These headaches come in clusters — appearing during several consecutive days, weeks, or months, and then disappearing, only to come back months or years later. Cluster headaches can come and go five or six times during a day. They're usually short-lived, lasting from 30 minutes to two or three hours each time.

  With a cluster headache, you may have a droopy-looking eyelid or sweating on the side that hurts, and you may find that moving around makes you feel better. Typically, cluster headaches aren't accompanied by nausea or vomiting. Pain comes from behind one eye. The eye may tear up or become red, and the nostril on this same side may run or feel congested.

Comparing migraines with auras to ones without

A relatively small percentage (about 20 percent) of migraine sufferers have the signals or symptoms called *auras* (visual disturbances, speech problems, distortions of smells and sounds, numb hands, feet, and lips). Some migraineurs have auras occasionally, while others have never had a single aura during their histories of headaches. (See more on auras in Chapter 2.)

Most migraineurs don't experience auras. So if your headaches don't come with auras, you aren't automatically placed in a different headache category (contrary to popular belief).

Looking at Some of the Reasons Why

If migraines run in your family, you may well have inherited a migraine tendency, which means that your gene pool set you up with a super-sensitive nervous system. Along with the hair you love and the nose you loathe, your predilection for migraines is part of your genetic material, and you can't run away from it. (Chapter 3 has more on the genetics/migraine connection.)

A migraine tendency is a dominant trait, so you probably inherited the penchant for having these headaches from your parent who suffers from migraines.

You may have noticed that certain foods, activities, sounds, or smells seem to trigger migraines. The problem is, this expected result may not occur every single time you eat Chinese food or take an aerobics class. It usually takes a village of triggers to raise a migraine: You never know if or when they're going to team up. (See food triggers in Chapter 11, exercise triggers in Chapter 12, environmental triggers in Chapter 13, and sleep-habit triggers in Chapter 14.)

Getting an Under-the-Hood Inspection and Tune Up

Diagnosing and treating migraines may require an investment of time, money, patience, trial-and-error, journaling (to discover triggers), and a strong working relationship with a doctor who does headache diagnosis.

Getting to the bottom of headaches can be complicated, so don't try to go it alone. If you do, chances are you'll flounder around for years without coming to any firm conclusions or finding painkillers that serve your needs. (See Chapter 6 on headache diagnosis.)

After you've been diagnosed with migraines, you can take your place as the Sultan of Scathing Headaches, starting to put remedies to work and implementing lifestyle changes. Find a positive tilt for the family and work issues associated with your headaches, and discover the best things to do when pain hits. You should also try to find ways to keep a migraine from forming.

Aspects of migraine management include: finding the right doctor and creating a treatment strategy, working to eliminate migraine triggers, handling family and work issues, and getting a heads-up on special issues, such as migraines associated with seniors, women, kids, stress, and sex. Plus, you need to familiarize yourself with red-flag headache signs that should send you scurrying to the emergency room.

Most of the time, migraines are quite manageable. Just figure out your headache triggers and rearrange certain aspects of your lifestyle, and you'll be on the road to sending your headaches to the B-team bench, where they'll languish and rarely take a starring role again.

Call on your top-flight patience when you start trying migraine treatments. Although you may get lucky and find that the first migraine drug your doctor recommends works perfectly for you, it's more common to have to go through a trial-and-error period of testing medications.

Migraines are quirky. If they weren't, doctors would be able to recommend the one super-sized honcho power-pill, and there would be no need for a book called *Migraines For Dummies*. But the truth is, migraine headaches come in as many varieties as there are materials in a fabric store. This variety makes them difficult — but certainly not impossible — to treat.

Handling Family and Work Issues

Getting a handle on family and work issues associated with migraines has several advantages. For one thing, you miss less work or school after you zero in on successful ways to manage your headaches. At the same time, though, the chronic nature of migraines means that you need to be prepared to deal with a headache that strikes when you're outside the home. You must have an arsenal of techniques ready to go.

Dealing with being misunderstood

Try real hard to understand all those folks who don't have migraines. You may wonder, "Why? What do you mean?" You may also feel indignant, "Hey, wait a minute — shouldn't I be the one expecting understanding?"

Well, the main reason you need to walk in others' shoes is because they definitely won't understand you or your headache predicament. Migraines are a strange illness to an outsider, and you really can't expect someone who hasn't had one to understand much about them. (See Chapter 24 for tips on dealing with people who don't get migraines.)

Most people who are migraine-free view migraine headaches in one or more of the following ways:

✔ **With skepticism:** They think that you're a hypochondriac.

✔ **With empathy:** They're sorry that you have to suffer.

✔ **With disinterest:** They don't want to hear about your migraines.

✔ **With anger:** They're mad when you have to cancel or call in sick, and your migraines inconvenience them.

✔ **With confusion:** Children, for example, have trouble understanding why a parent sometimes gets sick and can't do things for them, or why family activities have to be cancelled.

Taking these facts into consideration will help you deal with people around you in a happier, more consistent way. In return, you'll get better treatment because those close to you will know what to expect.

Also, the people skills involved in migraine management are extremely important because people who don't have migraines usually have trouble understanding them or relating to the sometimes-debilitating nature of headaches.

If head pain were your one-and-only problem, you'd be looking at a very different kind of malady. But the truth is, everyone associated with a migraineur is affected in some way (or to some degree) by the long-term nature of the affliction. It's up to you to set the tone for deft handling of your migraine's "extended family" of issues with all the people you deal with — family, friends, co-workers.

Basically, you either establish yourself as a capable, reliable individual who just happens to have headaches from time to time, or as a disabled person who wants everyone around her to jump when she needs help and show massive amounts of sympathy when she's down and out.

Exploring Options Galore

Without a doubt, the treatment/management situation today is very promising for migraine sufferers. You have much to celebrate. You have more options than your mother or grandmother had when they were nursing a headache. These options can help make your life easier and much more enjoyable.

The following advantages represent the final word on today's overall migraine picture:

- ✔ Doctors know much more about migraines than they did 20 years ago. The introduction of triptan migraine drugs, specifically, improved the migraine-treatment picture dramatically. (See prescription drugs in Chapter 8.)

- ✔ Healthcare providers take migraines seriously. They can guide migraine sufferers in eliminating lifestyle factors that can aggravate a highly sensitive nervous system. The upshot: The migraineur is able to become less dependent on medication.

- ✔ The drug options for treating migraines are head and shoulders above the ones that were available a few decades ago. (Today's medications are way more effective because some of them are migraine-specific.)

- ✔ Alternative therapies abound, and some of these may serve as excellent complements to your primary migraine management plan.

- ✔ Generally speaking, most people have more accepting attitudes about the severity of migraines, even though headaches remain shrouded in some degree of mystery.

- ✔ Migraine sufferers have found a voice. Most realize that they do, indeed, have a right to speak up and seek help.

Suffering in silence with a migraine has gone the way of pecking on a typewriter. Migraine treatment is now so smart and savvy that it represents multi-tasking at its best. Bill Gates would be proud. And you can be headache-free.

Chapter 2

Coping with the Symptoms

Migraines come in 31 original flavors, so take a number while you sort through the scads of symptoms and zillions of ideas on how to deal with your symptoms. In this chapter, we help you figure out what approaches provide migraine-relief, as well as things you can do to relieve the symptoms beyond the hammering pain. You also need to understand the causes of those cursed *rebound headaches* (headaches that are the result of overuse of medications), and what you can do to make sure that you never have one of those monsters again.

At any rate, while you're shopping around for answers for your migraines — measures that will keep them at bay or at least drop-kick them after they hit — you need an arsenal of quick fixes all poised and ready to fire.

Taking on the Big Three: Auras, Sensory Sensitivity, and Stomach Problems

The Big Three — auras, sensory sensitivity, and nausea — are the most common symptoms of migraines. Because you're reading *Migraines For Dummies* right now, chances are excellent that you already have some experience with this devilish trio.

Not all migraines come with auras. Moreover, not all migraines come with nausea and vomiting. These symptoms are, however, ones that many *migraineurs* (people who experience migraines) face.

Previewing an aura's light show

Visual and perceptual disturbances can accompany a migraine headache, and they do about 20 percent of the time. Typically, an aura starts about an hour before a migraine headache begins. You may hear or smell things that aren't really there. Some people experience numbness in their lips, hands, or feet, or have trouble speaking. Some theories on the causes of auras are: excitation of brain cells and decreased blood flow to the brain.

With different types of auras, you can experience

- Visual anomalies such as

  - White or colored squares, circles, or triangles that appear to be moving.

  - Zigzag lines around a dark center, shooting stars, or flashing lights.

  - Diminished field of vision (you see only half of your usual field) or blurriness.

Don't be afraid to describe your "sightings" when you're being evaluated by a doctor. You can be sure that neurologists and many other doctors are quite familiar with the strangeness of auras.

- Perceptional, physical, and other sensory anomalies

  - Distorted feelings about size. You may feel extremely small or super-sized.

  - Numbness in your face, lips, mouth, and/or hands.

- Dizziness or a spinning feeling.

- Food cravings or loss of appetite.

- Weakness, or feeling as if you're going to faint.

Usually lasting 20 to 40 minutes, auras typically come right before a headache — almost like the ding-ding-ding of a railroad-crossing bell, warning you that something big and scary is on its way. However, auras are also unpredictable. Just because they usually come before a headache doesn't mean that they can't pop up during the course of a migraine, too. In addition, you can also experience an aura but never get a headache. Sometimes, an aura lasts throughout a headache — particularly when it comes to increased sensitivity to light and sound. The intensity of auras range from being a minor annoyance to being an extremely frightening, hallucinogenic-type horror. Some migraineurs even say that they would accept the headache pain if they could bypass the aura.

Temporary visual disturbances can also occur with other medical conditions, such as retinal detachment (a serious eye problem that an *ophthalmologist* — an eye doctor — needs to evaluate immediately). Symptoms of retinal detachment are seeing flashing lights and having a sensation of a shade or curtain coming down over the vision in one eye.

By the way, in headache stages, the prodrome is the period preceding a headache. It's defined by warning signs such as dizziness, nausea, or aura. (For more information about headache staging, see Chapter 4.) The pro-drome stage has symptoms such as decreased appetite, fluid retention, irritability, and restlessness.

The type of headache that was once referred to as a *classic migraine* features an aura before the headache. Oddly enough, only a small percentage of migraine sufferers (about 10 to 20 percent) experience this "classic" symptom. In contrast, a *common migraine* doesn't feature an aura, yet the vast majority of migraineurs experience this aura-less migraine. Both of the terms — classic migraine and common migraine — are considered out-of-date. Now these headaches are currently referred to simply as *migraine with aura* and *migraine without aura.* Go figure.

Coping with sensitivity to light, smell, and sound

Your head is pounding, and you desperately want to get away from bright lights, bad smells, and loud noises. You feel as if this onslaught of hypersensitivity — common among migraineurs, by the way — is making your migraine pain a double- or triple-whammy. Some people report being bothered by only one or two of these, while others want to run from the entire offending trio of lights, smells, and sounds.

Lighting topics

Light sensitivity is such a common migraine symptom that it's in the top tier of symptoms and is usually a part of a migraine. Sensitivity can range from a mild reaction to a complete aversion to any kind of light. You may even experience bright lights as blinding pain. Fortunately, the light sensitivity has a simple remedy: Simply retreat to a dark room and lie down if necessary. If a dark room isn't an option, look for a spot with low light.

Smelling symptoms

Smells may bother you before or during a migraine. You may be ultra-sensitive to cooking odors. Sometimes you may even smell bad or pungent odors that don't exist. Your nose may run constantly, which may lead you to mistake your migraine for a sinus headache.

Finding perfumes and cigarette smoke very obnoxious isn't at all unusual for a migraine sufferer. Strong odors can actually make your pain worse, so try to steer clear of smells that are hard to handle. You can also try using an air purifier to neutralize problem odors or infusing a room with a pleasant and soothing smell, such as lavender.

Hearing hurts

Similar to finding smells bothersome, you may shudder when you hear noise. During a migraine, you may find that all kinds of sounds are unbearable. As is the case with staving off smells and lights, the remedy is simply a matter of getting away from the source of the problem.

Unfortunately, avoiding noise and insisting on quietness at home can throw a wet blanket on the atmosphere of your house. (For more on living with the ones you love and loathe when you have a migraine, head over to Chapter 17.) Some migraineurs use earplugs or ear protectors. But if having something on your head (protectors) accentuates the pain of your aching head, and you find earplugs annoying, these won't be viable solutions for you.

Combating stomach problems

You have a migraine plus the unwanted bonuses of nausea and vomiting. These stomach problems sometimes result from chemicals your brain releases during a migraine. Diarrhea and other changes in bowel habits can be troublesome, too. About half of all migraineurs experience stomach problems.

Migraine sufferers who are forced to cope with nausea and vomiting, along with head pain, usually can benefit from injections or suppositories that combat stomach woes. These aids work quickly and make you sleepy — which are both welcome effects. (Chapter 8 has more information on medications for nausea and vomiting.)

The only good thing that can be said about the nausea and vomiting that often accompany migraines is that this phase sometimes signals an easing of the head pain. On the other hand, for some folks, these stomach symptoms are only forerunners of the worst pain of the headache's entire course.

Other gastrointestinal problems you may experience at such times are: diarrhea, constipation, and stomach cramps. You may even find that your stomach has become almost paralyzed, which can cause you to have nausea and vomiting, rendering the oral medications that you take to improve the situation useless. This state of delayed emptying of the stomach is called *gastroparesis*. The upshot is that you need to resort to migraine medications via nasal spray, injection, or suppository.

Encountering Other Migraine Signs

Although the Big Three — auras, sensory sensitivity, and stomach problems — are the symptoms that tend to plague many migraineurs, other folks may have their own individual troublemakers. Symptoms are very erratic, and we don't have statistics on how many people experience which symptoms, but many people do have the Big Three plus some of the symptoms in the following list at some point:

- ✔ A drooping eyelid (more common in cluster headaches, but it can happen in migraines)
- ✔ A pale face or a flushed or very red face or a face that's extra sensitive
- ✔ A tender scalp
- ✔ Bloodshot eyes
- ✔ Blurred vision
- ✔ Cold hands and feet, or a feeling of being hot all over
- ✔ Dizziness or a feeling of spinning
- ✔ Food cravings or a total loss of appetite

Some migraine sufferers experience a personality switcharoo, showing three (or thirty) faces of Eve, and exhibiting raw and rugged personality traits. Feeling irritable and absolutely miserable, a migraineur can turn into a nasty creature who wants people out of his way, and then later wonders why he was so creepy.

If you're the one acting like your own evil twin, move away from people temporarily. On the other hand, if a migraine sufferer you know is showing his rough side, give him plenty of space. The good news is that this awfulness will end — just as soon as the headache subsides.

Using Quick Fixes as a Stopgap

Okay, so you're all in favor of this grand escapade we call migraine-busting. You have no problem with the idea of pulling out all the stops and nailing these wily little headache hooligans in 60 different ways.

Meanwhile, what's a guy to do about the pounding in his skull that's causing him grief so often and making it hard to get with the program of real life — as in, work, worship, socializing, and family?

What you need is a little parcel of quick-fix solutions to help you through the rough times while you're working on the long-term goal of migraine-busting.

Screech! Alrighty then. Here's the lowdown on how to relieve pain during your jaunt down the memory lane of the last of the big-time headaches. Try these lifestyle soothers:

✔ **Make sleep your new best friend.** Try to get the same amount of sleep each night, and strive for regularity in the times you go to bed and get up. Most people need seven or eight hours of sleep per night, but not everyone. Typically, when you can sleep as long as you want and wake up naturally, the number of hours you clock will be the amount that your body likes. Also, you must remember that getting about the same number of hours per night on weekends is important — or you may suffer a migraine from erratic sleep.

✔ **Use relaxation techniques.** Stress and anxiety can trigger headaches, so master skills that will empower you to decrease the toll that stress takes. Breathe deeply and meditate.

✔ **Massage your head.** When you feel a headache coming on, try the method that works for some migraineurs. Apply light pressure to your temples, your head, and the spot you feel pain radiating from.

✔ **Do low-key forms of exercise.** Slow jogging and brisk walking are good options. Pilates is excellent for stretching muscles and decreasing stress. In addition, many people get pain relief from practicing yoga. (See exercise recommendations in Chapter 12.)

✔ **Apply pressure to the right body points.** Find the tight and sore spots in your neck and shoulders, and press them firmly with your fingertips for several seconds. (Acupressure is addressed in Chapter 12.)

Some dietary upgrades that may help relieve pain or ward off migraines are

✔ **Drink plenty of water.** Get your water mojo going by downing eight to ten 8-ounce glasses a day. Dehydration can set the stage for a migraine.

Keep a quart (or liter) of bottled water on your desk, or somewhere handy, so you can avoid having to "guesstimate" your water intake. Drink this water during the day and then drink more water in the evening. If you're exercising a lot and sweating profusely, or if the weather's hot, increase the amount of water you drink, accordingly.

Don't make the mistake of saying, "Oh, I drink lots of tea and diet soda, so I get enough liquid." Those beverages are not water substitutes.

✔ **Set up a grazing plan.** Eat a number of very small meals/healthy snacks throughout the day, and never skip meals.

✔ **Eliminate alcohol.** Try decreasing and then eventually eliminating alcoholic beverages.

✔ **Stop smoking.** If you're not already participating in a smoking-cessation plan, find a hospital outpatient program that will help you achieve this critical health goal — or you can work with your doctor on a stop-smoking plan.

✔ **Purify your diet:** Eat fruits, vegetables, and other natural foods, and avoid foods with preservatives and MSG (monosodium glutamate). (See food triggers in Chapter 11.)

When you use any kind of migraine medication (over-the-counter or prescription), make sure that you don't take it more than two days a week. If this medication schedule leaves you in pain, talk to your doctor and get advice on what to do. Avoid the fly-by-the-seat-of-your-pants approach to self-medicating. This tactic takes the "listen to your body" adage to a place you don't want to go.

Keep your optimism at a fever pitch while you're on your migraine-busting mission. You definitely can find your way toward a higher plateau, where you can live more peacefully and less painfully. Migraineurs do it all the time.

Chapter 3

Knowing Your Foes

. . . .

. . . .

*W*hen head monsters are pounding nails into your neurons, you're ready to try anything. Before you grab a random remedy, however, try developing a headache-busting agenda where you check out the usual suspects. Start by creating a journal in which you keep up with the foods you eat and your lifestyle habits — all the time looking for problem areas that seem to contribute to headache evolution.

Doing a little detective work can help you zero in on your personal troublemakers. Certain aspects of your meals and your environment may be headache-causing "toxins," so the sooner you pinpoint these triggers, the quicker you can get a handle on the fate of your pain.

Keeping a Journal to Discover Reasons and Triggers

Who knew? You probably never figured that some day you'd be sitting in your living room with a spiral notebook or a handheld computer, making notes about the things you do, eat, smell, and hear on a quest to discover the weasels behind your migraines. If you prefer a ready-to-go itemizer: Copy the journal in Figure 3-1.

Headache Journal

Onset and Duration	Headache Traits	Possible Triggers	Remedies and Their Effectiveness
Date of headache: Time since last headache: number of hours, days or weeks: Where were you when you got the headache: Signs that a headache was coming: visual disturbances, yawning, drowsiness, and so on. List all: Duration of headache: number of hours or days:	**Associated symptoms:** nausea, vomiting, light or sound sensitivity, and so on. List all: **Pain rating** on a scale of 1 (very little pain) to 10 (incapacitating pain): **Location of pain:** on side of the head, both sides, generalized, behind the eye, and so on. List all: **Type of pain:** throbbing, dull ache, sharp, band-like. List all: Does movement aggravate your headache? Is the pain: off and on or consistent?	**Emotions:** List anything especially exciting or anxiety-producing: **Hormones:** Indicate whether your headache was before, during, or after your period, and whether you're menopausal: **Food and drink:** List what you ate and drank. Include caffeine consumption and whether you consumed your usual amount at the usual time: **Alcohol/drug consumption:** List any alcohol or drugs you ingested: **Physical activity:** List what type of exercise you engaged in, including whether you had sex: **Environment:** Were you exposed to excessive sunlight or bright light: a change in the weather, a change in altitude, dust, smoke, and so on. List all:	**Remedies Tried** **Over-the-counter medication:** Advil, Excedrin, aspirin, and so on. List type and dosage: **Prescription medication:** List name and dosage: **Complementary remedies:** List method and how long you used it: How far into the headache did you try the treatment? **Effectiveness** **Medication:** Indicate, in hours, how long it took the medication to be effective, as well as whether it dulled the pain but didn't eliminate it, or didn't help at all: **Complementary remedy:** Indicate what effect the remedy had on your head pain and on your ability to cope with your migraine:

Figure 3-1: Sharing your headache journal can help your doctor treat your migraines.

Whatever method you use to journal, the important step is to launch an intensive search for the Trigger Terrors that get together and conspire against you. These triggers are the ones that begin the trek down the road that leads to the mega-pain of a migraine headache.

When starting a journal, follow these basic steps:

1. **Carry your journal at all times.**

2. **Record what you eat, where you go, what the environment's like, and so on.**

   Check out Figure 3-1 for all the specifics of what you should jot down in your headache journal.

3. **Write down the specifics of any migraine — when it started, what it felt like, and so on — and the pattern of the pain you experience.**

   A pain pattern could be a migraine that occurs every four to five days and lasts about three hours each time, for example.

4. **Note the remedies you try and how effective they are.**

Journaling may strike you as time-consuming and, well, maybe a little bit *boring*. . . . but hey, if it can put you back in the Game of Life, feeling good and rambunctious (with a head free of pain), it has to be well worth the minutes you devote to jotting down your pain patterns and possible triggers.

A *trigger* is anything, whether internal or external, that sets a migraine attack in motion. Typically, you make a judgment call when identifying a trigger (is it a trigger or not?); after all, suspected triggers don't wear banners that say, "Hey, we're here to mess with you!" Plus, a specific trigger may not cause a headache every single time — instead, a specific combination of factors may be the catalyst.

At the end of each day, make a notation next to any item in your journal that seems to contribute to the development of a headache within 30 minutes to an hour. Track four or five separate headache days. Remember, things that seem to be triggers may actually only be coincidences; recording a number of headaches helps narrow things down.

Understanding Inherited Migraines

You have beautiful turquoise eyes from your father, straight teeth from your grandmother, and an incredible singing voice from your grandfather — and, well, migraine headaches from your mother. (Of course, she feels really bad about it. But still, that little tag-you're-it came floating down in the gene pool when you were trolling for a set of traits, and now it's pretty much a done deal.) How can you inherit migraines? Well, nothing's truly set in stone on the migraine story, but many experts believe that a specific gene determines a person's proclivity for migraines.

A genetic predisposition for migraines in certain people appears to be a given. In fact, most migraineurs have a strong family history of agonizing head pain. Underscoring the theory of inheriting migraines is researchers' discovery of an area on chromosome 19 that relates to a certain kind of migraine. This finding points to a specific inherited pattern in families who have *hemiplegic migraine.* This headache types causes temporary paralysis on one side of the body. The paralysis, which occurs in your face, arm, or leg, can last from one hour to days, but it usually lasts for about 24 hours. You can't distinguish this weakness or paralysis from a stroke, so you need to be evaluated by a doctor who can consider all causes of acute onset weakness. (Check out Chapter 4 for a run-through of the different types of headaches.)

You can inherit familial hemiplegic migraine if your family tree has at least two people who have migraines with aura that feature this one-sided weakness. (For more information about migraines with aura, see Chapter 2.) So you may inherit the *tendency* to have migraines, but it takes your own personal trigger (or two or three) to set off a headache. Researchers regard the migraine tendency as a dominant trait. If one of your parents has migraines, you may inherit the proclivity. You're more likely to inherit it from your mother than your father.

A less common theory is that everyone in the world has the potential for migraines, but some people have a low threshold to triggers, whereas others have a high threshold. If you're a low-threshold type, your migraines trigger more easily than those of the high-threshold type.

Checking Your Environment for Allergens

Headache sufferers can be supersensitive to the content of their environments, so evaluating your own home and workplace for possible headache triggers is a good idea. (See Chapter 13 for more detail about the role the environment plays in triggering headaches.)

The following list provides some general tips for improving your environment:

- ✔ Clean your indoor air by placing a negative-ion generator in your bedroom.
- ✔ Change air-conditioner filters frequently.

✔ Set houseplants around your rooms to filter indoor pollution. Plants that horticulturists recommend for filtering air include aloe vera, ficus, philodendron, spider plants, and areca palms.

✔ Have your tap water tested for impurities and carcinogens.

✔ Install a home water-purification unit or have bottled water delivered to your home.

✔ Check into the indoor air quality of places you frequent, such as your workplace (see Chapter 13 for more on testing indoor air quality).

✔ Hire an inspector to check your home for mold, pollens, bacteria, asbestos, radon, elevated levels of carbon monoxide, leaky gas furnaces, and noxious fumes.

Finding Dietary Villains

Diet is a category that can make a major difference in the frequency and severity of your headaches. Most people who suffer from migraines have one or more triggers in the food-and-beverage genre. You just have to figure out which ones are yours. (See Chapter 11 for common culprits.)

Recording everything you eat and drink enables you to key in on the food/drink ogres that give you fits, so be sure that you don't leave out anything. Food and other things you ingest that may cause migraines include

✔ Beverages, including alcohol, coffee, tea, and so on

✔ Foods you eat on the road (in the car, at movies, at friends' and relatives' homes)

   When recording food triggers, most people don't include road foods, because they think that they have no control over what they eat away from home.

✔ Meals and snacks

✔ Medications (prescription and over-the-counter), including hormone replacement therapy and birth control pills

✔ Vitamins

Poor eating habits, such as failing to drink enough fluids (which can cause dehydration) and skipping meals, can also cause problems.

Figure 3-2 shows some of the more common migraine triggers.

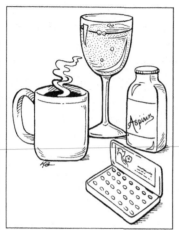

Figure 3-2:
Caffeine, redwine, over-the-counter medications, and birth control pills can all trigger migraines.

Leaving behind the dark, sweet stuff (reality therapy for chocoholics)

Here's the latest theory from the chocolate folks: After experts told us for decades that the dark, delicious stuff called chocolate was a migraine trigger, it has been determined that it's not true, after all. As Emily Litella used to say on *Saturday Night Live*: "Never mind!" Unfortunately, we can line up a number of migraineurs who beg to disagree. For them, it does indeed seem to trigger headaches.

You have to make your own call. Go ahead and dip into that box of chocolates if you just can't resist — but go into it with your eyes wide open. Truth be told, sometimes a food is so delicious that the taste-temptation payoff is almost worth the headache. Almost. But not quite.

As a general rule, if you're thrashing about for answers to your migraines, it may be smart to eliminate chocolate for a while. If you find out that chocolate is not a trigger, you can always return to chocoholic heaven.

Checking for MSG on menus and labels

Here at the outset of migraine-busting, you need to know that one of the most common food triggers for migraine-prone folks is *MSG (monosodium glutamate),* a flavor enhancer often added to Chinese foods and also found in seasoning salt and other flavor enhancers. Years ago, cooks commonly added MSG to veggies to jazz them up (the stuff perks up the taste of food). But soon those little shakers of MSG became less in demand, as more and more people began to link migraines to MSG. The bad rap was well deserved, and, like a nickname, it stuck.

If you find that MSG does trigger your migraine headaches, become a good label reader. Develop a habit of checking for it in foods you buy, and be vigilant for other camouflaged words that let MSG sneak into your foods; some common aliases for MSG include sodium glutamate, hydrolyzed protein, calcium caseinate, and sodium caseinate.

Some of the many places MSG may hide include the following:

✔ Asian foods in supermarkets

✔ Candy and gum

✔ Canned soups

✔ Chinese food in restaurants

✔ Dry-roasted nuts

✔ Flavorings such as soy sauce, broth, and bouillon

✔ Frozen dinners

✔ Iced tea mixes

✔ Meats packaged with sauces (sometimes)

✔ Packaged gravy

✔ Processed meats

✔ Some sports drinks and diet drinks

✔ Spices/seasonings

Zeroing in on Exercises that Make Your Head Hurt

You take a step aerobics class and end up paying for it with a migraine. You notice a trend: Every time you exercise vigorously, your head hurts afterward. Yes, exercise can trigger migraines in some folks, but don't give up on being a fitness enthusiast just because you've had some bad experiences. In fact, exercise can actually be used to help fend off headaches. You simply have to figure out which forms of exercise work for you and which forms trigger headaches.

Regular exercise three times a week for 30 to 45 minutes may actually ward off painful headache episodes. Movement increases your brain's production of *endorphins* — those well-known (and much talked about) chemical schmoozers that are both mood elevators and pain reducers.

If you suspect that exercise is a migraine trigger for you, list in your journal the length of time it takes you warm up, the type of exercise you use, the duration of your workout, and how soon after the workout you develop a headache.

Just keep in mind that the key element of a migraine sufferer's workout should be a slow stretch-and-move warm-up prior to cutting loose.

Abandoning oh-that's-intense exercises

So, you love Spinning (an exercise where you pedal a stationary bike from low to high speeds to simulate uphill and downhill riding), or you can't get enough of the high-energy bench class at your health club, but you always walk away with a headache. *Hello!* These exercises are triggers for you!

The key word here is "acceptance." You simply can't get your heart set on defining yourself as a super Spinner, an ace aerobics performer, or a champion triathlete if doing these workouts gives you grief (headaches) on a consistent basis.

Bypassing known terrors for kinder forms of exercise

The good news is that there are many kinds of exercises you *can* do. Use them as replacements for the tough-to-handle workouts that lead to headaches.

Try participating in a water exercise class or a low-impact aerobics class. Both are widely available at YMCAs, YWCAs, and health clubs. (See Chapter 12 for more exercise options.)

Start a program of walking, swimming, yoga, Pilates, dance, or cycling. Sometimes you can make the pain go away by doing some slow-motion exercising when you feel the first twinges of a headache.

Hydration is extra-important for exercisers who have a tendency to get migraines. Have your water bottle handy, and keep track of how much water you drink so you can make sure that you're getting enough. (Most days, you should drink about eight to ten 8-ounce glasses of water. Increase that amount by one glass per hour of vigorous, sweat-inducing exercise.)

Sure, all that super-imbibing will have you trotting to the bathroom more often, but it's a small price to pay for staying headache-free.

Keying in on Other Migraine Triggers

So many triggers, so little time. But somehow your body is willing to work overtime in an effort to scrounge up gnarly reactions to many of the ordinary elements of everyday living.

So even if you're perfectly immune to most food and exercise triggers, don't start feeling too smug. A migraine thug may be waiting right around the corner, and you'll be in for big trouble when that trigger-happy thing stomps across your brain, toting a cartful of ammo.

Sometimes even old friends seem to turn on you. Nontriggers convert to triggers — or at least, that's what you think is happening. Things that you have always tolerated well — medications, foods, exercise — get rebellious and go toxic one day for no apparent reason. So you're shocked when you develop a headache as an almost immediate response to something that you've lived in harmony with for years. Unfair and nonsensical! Yes, you're right on both counts — but it happens nonetheless.

The truth is, this is what probably happens in such cases: You have an onslaught of triggers act together to cause a migraine — so it just *seems like* something benign and nontrigger-like is suddenly giving you pain.

Migraineurs report that the following things sometimes trigger migraines:

- Bright lights
- Cigarette or cigar smoke
- Environmental changes: weather, heat, cold
- Fatigue or hangover
- Menopause or perimenopause (see Chapter 19)
- Menstrual cycle (see Chapter 19)
- Puberty
- Sexual activity (see Chapter 21)
- Sleep disturbances: restlessness, insomnia
- Sleep patterns: uneven sleeping, getting up and going to bed at different times, and a wide range in the number of hours you sleep (see Chapter 14)

✔ Smells and sounds

✔ Surgery/anesthesia

✔ Travel

✔ Worries, anxiety, stress (see Chapter 22)

Most people have triggers. For you, the question is "How many of these triggers have to team up in order to cause a migraine?" You may tiptoe past triggers all the time, and they don't make themselves known as bugaboos as long as you're still hovering below your threshold. Your head gets a full frontal attack only when your body's forces get overwhelmed by enemies packing enormous pain bolts. In other words, it often takes a village of triggers to raise a headache.

If it's not one thing, it's another

Remember when Gilda Radner played the woe-ridden, jaw-chewing Roseanne Roseannadanna character, whose motto was "it's always something!" on *Saturday Night Live*?

You have to figure that she (or one of the show's comedy writers) had migraines — because, when it comes to migraines, it's always something. And, if it's not one thing, it's another.

A college freshman told us that she didn't understand why Chinese food would give her a headache one time after she ate it, not have an affect on her the next time she ate it, and then have an affect on her again the third time. The matter got really confusing one night when she ate chocolate, which she nibbled frequently, and then got a horrible migraine. Until she ate that particular dessert (chocolate mousse), chocolate had never been a problem for her! Did the chocolate have a bad reaction with her birth control pills or the acetaminophen she had been taking all day?

Then she read an article about how triggers can team up to cause migraines. While one thing alone (chocolate, for example) may not be enough to spur a headache, several together may do the job. Until that point, she had worried that some things could just turn into demons overnight, leaving behind a killer headache for her to exorcise. Basically, what she called a "chocolate migraine" was really the result of a bunch of triggers forming a powerful posse and giving her head a wallop she'd never forget.

This young woman talked to her gynecologist, who had firsthand experience with migraine headaches. The doctor told her that triggers are so unpredictable sometimes, that it seems as if a perfectly friendly thing (tea or peanut butter) will suddenly sprout a devil's tail — and you end up with a really splitting headache that sends you to bed to sleep it off. The doctor also explained how sometimes certain things will bother you (and start a headache), and other times, they won't. "They have to get together with some buddies — other triggers — to cause a migraine, but all too often, that happens."

The doctor told her to track her food and lifestyle triggers in a headache journal. A few weeks later, she took her journal back to the doctor and got a prescription for a migraine medication that really helped her. In two hours, it knocked out a migraine! So she discovered that trigger-tracking was well worth the effort and time.

Stopping Triggers in their Tracks

Several lifestyle issues can influence the severity and frequency of your headaches. Make sure you follow these guidelines:

✔ Stay far, far away from red wine, aged cheeses (especially sharp cheddar), and caffeinated coffee. (The latter is a problem because trying to go cold turkey when kicking caffeine can give you withdrawal headaches, and if you're predisposed to migraines, you can bet that your headaches will be killer.) Taper off caffeine intake over a period of a week or so. (See Chapter 11 for more foods to avoid.)

✔ Don't smoke.

✔ Get plenty of rest. Don't sleep 12 hours a night, but don't get exhausted to the gills, either. The right amount of rest varies with each individual; you can often tell what your body requires by checking the number of hours you sleep naturally, when no alarm or person wakes you up. For some people, it may be six hours — for others, it may be eight or nine.

✔ Bump up the fiber content of your diet (more whole-grain cereals and breads, and veggies). See Chapter 11 for diet tips.

✔ Eat very few fat- or sugar-laden foods.

✔ Get enough calcium and magnesium. Every day, you need about 1,200 mg of calcium and 300 mg of magnesium. (If your diet is deficient in these, you can use vitamin supplements.)

Doctors see low magnesium levels in women who are on birth control pills, are having PMS symptoms, or are taking estrogen-only hormone replacement for menopause. Studies show a link between low magnesium and migraines in men and women. Some researchers even go so far as to suggest that the root of all migraine evil is a deficiency of magnesium.

✔ Avoid migraine triggers such as alcohol, chocolate, artificial sweeteners, concentrated sugar, pickled foods, MSG (monosodium glutamate — a flavor enhancer), cured meats (with nitrates), sulfites, olives, snow peas, and pickles. (See Chapter 11.) Sulfites are found in maraschino cherries, instant potatoes, frozen french fries, shredded coconut, dried fruits, syrups, soup mixes, vegetable juices, fruit juices, lemon juice, wine, raisins, and pizza. MSG is often in Chinese foods, processed meats, tenderizers, canned and processed foods, and soy sauce.

✔ Laugh.

✔ Meditate.

✔ Walk or work out regularly — but don't turn into a workout fanatic. Over-exercising can decrease estrogen. As with everything, try the moderation route. (And be sure to warm up before workouts.)

Triggers get together and party hearty

Here's how triggers wreak havoc:

Let's say that you know alcohol always gives you a headache, but one night at a friend's wedding reception, you just can't resist a glass of champagne. (You're dying to be "normal," so you make a toast and chug-a-lug the bubbly.)

Ah-hah! No migraine! *Whoa!* You're impressed. This is a sign. An omen. It must mean that you've finally outgrown that irksome alcohol trigger altogether, right? Wrong.

What it means is that when wine, champagne, or a mixed drink gave you a headache in the past, the drink had some partners in crime. You drank it on a day when other factors were working their black magic — you were about to start your menstrual period, you just finished a 12-hour work day, or you skipped lunch. Or all three.

Avoiding food triggers judiciously is one of the smartest things a migraine sufferer can do to help herself.

Instead of drinking alcohol when you know you'll be sorry you did, drown your disappointment in white wedding cake or cute groomsmen (or bridesmaids).

Part II
Getting Diagnosed

The 5th Wave
By Rich Tennant

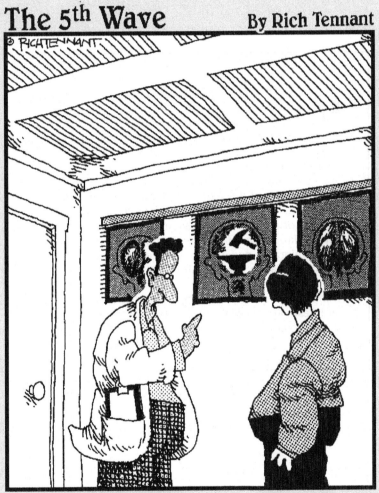

"Initially I was going to say your migraines were caused by a hormonal trigger to the hypothalamus. But this X-ray indicates you actually have a tiny hammer striking an anvil in your head."

In this part . . .

You're leaving behind the days of thinking that you finally figured out your headaches, only to read a magazine article that changes your mind, and bam! — you're back to square one.

The focus of Part II is a once-and-for-all conclusion: Your doctor will help you separate your migraine headaches from the other types of headaches even though symptoms can overlap and confuse the diagnosis. It's crucial to have a good migraine doc on board to help determine what kind of headache you actually have.

At the doctor's office, you have your head examined, find out if tests are needed to verify the diagnosis, and get tips on how to come up with your own migraine-management plan.

Chapter 4

Distinguishing a Migraine from Other Head Pain

*T*o fight the good fight, you must know your enemy. The biggest problem with headache-sorting is that people mistakenly think that they have migraines when their headaches are of a different type, or they don't think that they have migraines when they actually do. It's a wild, wild world out there in Headacheland, and figuring out your skull signals is the first step to taming your migraine headaches.

This chapter helps you get up close and personal with different types of headaches to find out whether you have bona-fide migraines. We clue you in to symptoms of the various types of headaches.

By the time you're through with this chapter, you'll be madly conversant in headache-speak and amazingly savvy about the headache universe.

To get in on the New Day of Migraine Management, you need to first look at the different types of headaches and the physiological path of migraines. This information paves your way to the next step — getting your doctor's help in figuring out whether your head pain fits the migraine mold or is the result of another type of headache or health condition. After you determine what is causing your headaches, you'll be ready to zero in on the best treatments.

Sorting Headache Types

Sorting out the different types of headaches is a good first step for determining what's giving you head pain. In the following sections, we lay out the various classes and types of headaches so that you can know your enemy.

Ranking primary and secondary headaches

Generally speaking, headaches fall into two categories: primary (the headache as the problem) and secondary (the headache as a symptom of an organic disease). With *primary headaches,* the headache itself is the big, bad Goliath causing your symptoms. When you have a primary migraine headache, you can't blame anything but the alpha dog — the migraine. Migraines are primary headaches. With *secondary headaches,* the headache is one of the symptoms caused by another medical condition. A headache caused by meningitis is an example of a secondary headache.

Headaches are also categorized as either episodic or chronic. *Episodic headaches* are headaches that you have now and then. Headaches are considered *chronic headaches* if you have them for more than 15 days per month. The conventional wisdom suggests that most chronic headaches stem from sinus disease, eye problems, or allergies. The fact is that most people who suffer from chronic headaches have migraine or tension-type headaches — and few of these folks have other health problems that contribute to their headaches.

Headaches can be especially hard to diagnose, because they often have conflicting symptoms. The following traits show the chameleon nature of headaches:

- Headaches can mutate from one type to another.
- You may suffer from more than one type of headache.
- Your headache type may fit into two categories at the same time.

All of these traits can apply to migraines as well as to other types of headaches. The following sections deal specifically with migraines and how to differentiate them from other headaches.

Spotting migraine impersonators

Because many people automatically think that a bad headache is a migraine, it's easy for all types of headaches to be mistakenly labeled migraines. This confusion can be dangerous if you have a brain hemorrhage and you treat it as though it's a migraine. The improper treatment can result in a potentially fatal delay in getting help.

Another danger in treating a headache as though it's a migraine is that you may take the wrong medication. Some drugs are headache-specific. In other words, certain medications work best on cluster headaches, some target tension-type headaches, and others are migraine-specific (see Chapter 8 for more on migraine medications).

Ah, clearly a migraine by any other name would still be . . . yes, a migraine. But headaches can only be considered migraines if they come with the unique characteristics of migrainehood. You need to get acquainted with the headbangers that only masquerade in the guise of the Big M, but are really cluster or tension-type renegades. Their symptoms are no picnic, mind you, but these migraine impersonators shouldn't be mistaken for a true migraine.

If you have bad headaches that aren't migraines, you may have tension-type headaches or, much less likely, cluster headaches (see the following sections for more on tension-type and cluster headaches). If these shoes don't fit, you may have one of the off-the-wall varieties of headache (see "Visiting the other headaches," later in this chapter).

The following headache characteristics are signals that you probably don't have a migraine:

- ✔ Your pain is a dull ache without any throbbing.
- ✔ Your shoulders and neck muscles feel knotted-up.
- ✔ You get a headache only after exercise or sex.
- ✔ Your headaches are getting steadily worse.

   This symptom may be a sign of an *organic headache* — a headache caused by a problem such as an abnormality in the brain or skull. An abnormality may be a brain aneurysm, a brain tumor, a hematoma, meningitis, a brain infection or abscess, encephalitis, or a cerebral hemorrhage.

Encapsulating the cluster headache

By looking at the traits of the other headaches that may be mistaken for migraines, you can detect the differences and key into the type that you actually have. For example, cluster headaches, which are often even more painful than migraines, are rare. They frequently occur at night, and they target men more often than women. The following symptoms can indicate a cluster headache:

- ✔ You have a sudden, piercing pain on one side of your head.
- ✔ You have a cluster of symptoms. You may have pain behind one eye on one side of your head; your eye (on the pain side) may become red and

tear up; your eyelid may droop; and your nostril on the pain side may feel congested or runny.

✔ You have several headaches per day over a period of weeks or months. Because headache attacks group up, the name "cluster" is used to describe them.

✔ Your headaches last 30 to 90 minutes (or a few hours).

Some researchers contend that cluster headaches reflect a dysfunction of your brain's *hypothalamus* (the portion of the brain that secretes substances that control various body functions). Another hypothesis is that your neck arteries are feeding incorrect amounts of oxygen and carbon dioxide to your brain by way of your blood.

Cluster headaches respond well to medication. Another popular treatment is oxygen therapy, where you're zapped with oxygen through a facemask. The oxygen can get rid of your pain if the treatment takes place early in an attack.

Cluster headaches can be like stormy rain clouds. They move around, they sprinkle darkness here and there, and they show up now and then. Your headache goes away and then pops up again later the same day. Some people report having as many as eight headaches in a single day!

One type of headache similar to cluster headaches is chronic paroxysmal hemicrania. Lasting about 10 to 20 minutes, this headache has a tendency to come and go many times in a given day. *Paroxysms* refer to stabbing pains happening in rapid succession, usually around the eye area. *Hemicranial* means "half of the head," or a one-sided pain. Combine the two and you have stabbing pains on one side of the head that are chronic (experienced periodically over a long period of time). About half of people with severe migraines have one-sided pain, but if you have this symptom with chronic paroxysmal hemicrania, it's likely that a doctor will recommend an MRI (see Chapter 6), because it can be a sign that a tumor or abnormal blood vessel is causing your headaches. If you have chronic paroxysmal hemicrania, you may have this type of headache off and on for several years.

Untangling tension-type headaches

Tension-type headaches are as common as dirt. These headaches are the kind that anyone can experience at pretty much any time. You feel the pain, all right, but tension-type headaches typically respond fairly quickly to pain medication — ibuprofen or acetaminophen — or physical therapy, such as neck and shoulder exercises or massage.

For some tension-type headache sufferers, learning better stress-handling techniques (see Chapter 9) and eliminating triggers can help alleviate their headaches.

When tension-type headaches are episodic (occurring randomly), they can usually be relieved with over-the-counter (OTC) medications. But if you take medication almost daily for your headaches, see a doctor, because you're probably having chronic tension-type headaches. (Your headaches may be chronic if you're having them most days, and the trend has been in place for months.)

You may get a tension-type headache because you tense up when you're under stress — if this is the case, your headache stems from muscle tension. Or you may get tension-type headaches when you're hungry or exhausted.

The following conditions are suspected causes of chronic tension-type headaches:

- ✔ Abnormalities in the brain's pain control system
- ✔ Abnormalities of the neck muscles, bones, or jaw
- ✔ Depression
- ✔ Emotional factors, such as worry, dread, fear, and excitement
- ✔ Eyestrain
- ✔ Fatigue
- ✔ Misaligned teeth
- ✔ Poor posture
- ✔ Stress

Don't be confused by the word "tension." Tension isn't always the cause of this type of headache.

If your headaches are the tension-type, you have some of the following symptoms:

- ✔ Your skull feels tender, and your headache can be characterized as a dull, constant ache that's mild or moderate on the pain scale.
- ✔ You feel a pressure or bandlike sensation around the upper area of both sides of your head (as if you're wearing a headband that's five sizes too small), or the back of your head hurts.
- ✔ Your neck and shoulder muscles feel tightly knotted.
- ✔ You don't vomit, get nauseated, or have visual disturbances (in contrast to some migraines).
- ✔ The pain creeps up slowly.

Usually, you get these headaches during times of high stress, but you may also have the same type of headache on a day without stress.

If you have tension-type headaches all the time (the kind that people call "sick headaches"), you may be the unlucky recipient of the dynamic duo — coexisting migraine and tension-type headaches. This combination is also called a *transformed migraine.* The tension/migraine pairing comes with varied symptoms that befit its hybrid nature. People who have coexisting migraine and tension-type headaches often overuse medications because they experience day-to-day head pain. The overuse of medication can induce rebounding problems (see "Recoiling from Rebound Headaches," later in this chapter) and cause individual migraine attacks to evolve into chronic daily headaches.

Visiting the other headaches

The miscellaneous headache group is interesting because of its utter diversity. And it just keeps on growing — even as we speak.

The miscellaneous group continues to grow because headaches are such rugged individualists. They come in almost as many shapes and patterns as fingerprints. When researchers, physicians, and headache sufferers discover new types of headaches, they just slap new names on them. Some of these names eventually make their way into the medical terminology for headaches.

There are too many miscellaneous headaches to list all of them here, so the following list just describes a few of the types in this category. (By the way, the word "benign" in the first three examples contrasts the headaches with their evil-twin versions that are more serious.)

- **Benign cough headache:** Coughing, sneezing, lifting things, or straining with a bowel movement are all actions that can bring on benign cough headache. The pain is usually located on both sides of the head, and it can last anywhere from seconds to a few minutes. Benign cough headache is most common in men, but overall, it's rare. Before the diagnosis can be made, the doctor must do an exam and run tests to exclude problems such as a tumor.

- **Benign exertion headache:** Physical activity triggers a headache that sometimes (but not always) evolves into a migraine. This headache usually occurs during or after prolonged exertion, or with intense bursts of activity. Because benign exertion headaches sometimes evolve into migraines, they're also referred to as *exertion migraines.*

  Typically, the pain is throbbing. Activities that can trigger benign exertion headaches include coughing, running, lifting things, and bending over. To treat benign exertion headaches, stop the activity that triggers your headache and take acetaminophen.

In rare cases, when the pain is sudden and severe after exertion, the headache can signal a hemorrhage inside the head (one cause of a thunderclap headache, which is covered later in this list). So if you have any doubt about your exertion headaches, go to the emergency room (ER) and have a doctor explore your aching head.

- **Benign sexual headache:** This type of headache is commonly diagnosed in people who are middle-aged. It occurs during or after sexual intercourse.

  To confirm that your headaches are truly benign, you need to be evaluated by your physician to make sure that they aren't caused by serious conditions, such as a brain hemorrhage or lesion. (See Chapter 21.)

- **Cold stimulus headache:** Also called an *ice-cream headache,* this one hits when you consume a cold drink or cold food. It usually lasts just a minute or two.

- **Decompression headache:** Rapid *decompression* (a change in the pressure of gases that your body is accustomed to) can cause nitrogen gas bubbles to form in your tissues and blood. The gas bubbles can result in headaches and even more serious problems. Decompression headaches are primarily diagnosed in divers and pilots. The decompression headache is sometimes referred to as an *airplane headache.*

- **Drug-withdrawal headache:** This type of headache occurs when you stop the chronic use of a drug (including caffeine).

- **External compression headache:** This type of headache results from continued external pressure on the head (such as from swim goggles or a tight hat). External compression headaches are sometimes referred to as *swim-goggle headaches.*

- **Glaucoma-related headache:** Glaucoma is an eye problem that can cause a bad headache. When you have an acute glaucoma attack, you may see halos around lights or experience blurred vision. You may also suffer from a headache, extreme eye and forehead pain, vomiting, and red eye. To safeguard your vision, see an eye doctor (ophthalmologist) as soon as possible if you think that your headaches may be caused by glaucoma.

- **Hangover headache:** You drink too much, and you're struck with a headache the next day (or the same day). Take a headache pill of the over-the-counter variety and bypass the hair-of-the-dog remedy.

- **High-altitude headache:** This type of headache typically occurs within 24 hours of going to an altitude above 10,000 feet. The best treatment: Descend to a lower altitude. Medications can also be effective.

- **Idiopathic stabbing headache:** This type of headache is characterized by a one-sided, dull, aching pain combined with a recurring, sharp, ice-pick-like pain. (This headache could down an elephant!) The cause of this headache type is unknown. You may also hear this type of headache referred to as a *jabs-and-jolts headache* or a *stab jab headache*. These are common in people with migraines. However, if you have this type of headache with growing frequency, see your doctor for evaluation.

✔ **Low-blood-sugar headache:** You skipped a meal or didn't eat enough, and the result is an easy-to-trace headache. Take an over-the-counter medication and eat something. Of course, even gobbling down food won't necessarily stop the chain reaction that has already been set in motion. Make sure that you don't skip your next meal. Throwing off your body's fuel clock by skipping meals is never a good thing for a migraine-sensitive system like yours.

✔ **Occipital neuralgia:** This is a headache characterized by sudden, stabbing pains in the back of the head. You may also have tenderness in the same area. Pain in the back of your head can be related to migraine or tension-type headaches or organic diseases.

✔ **Post-seizure headache:** Following a generalized seizure, it's believed that cerebral blood vessels dilate, often resulting in a generalized headache.

✔ **Post-surgery or post-injury headache:** If neck or head tissue is repositioned or affected significantly during surgery or a head or neck injury, the result can be a splitting headache.

✔ **Sinus headache:** With this headache type, your swollen, irritated sinuses make your poor head hurt. An allergy or a cold can often cause a sinus headache. Your head pain, which often follows a sinus-blocking upper respiratory infection, hammers right above or below your eyes.

People who have chronic sinus disease usually don't have headaches. Sinus headaches are more likely to occur with acute sinusitis. You can treat a sinus headache with antibiotics (if you have a sinus infection) or decongestants.

Sometimes doctors find that people aren't sure where their sinuses are. In case you're hazy on the location of your sinuses, they're found under your cheekbone on each side, under your forehead bone, and behind your nose. (When sinuses get inflamed, your head can hurt.)

✔ **Thunderclap headache:** This type is characterized by the sudden onset of a very intense headache. Consider these headaches a warning sign to go to the ER immediately, because thunderclap headaches can be caused by conditions as serious as a ruptured *aneurysm* (ballooning of the wall of a blood vessel) or *subarachnoid hemorrhage* (bleeding in the brain).

✔ **TMJ headache:** Temporomandibular joint syndrome (TMJ) may be better known for its clicking, popping jaw-joint sounds, but it's also a cause of big, bad headaches. Grinding your teeth at night adds to the problem.

✔ **Travel headache:** Those car trips that make you motion-sick can sometimes result in major-league headaches. Get rid of your headache by taking acetaminophen and getting out of the car. You can also use a preventive motion-sickness medication in advance (about 30 minutes before you get in the car).

✔ **Weekend headache:** On the weekend, you wake up late with an awful headache — probably stemming from not having had your morning dose of coffee (caffeine) at the regular time (earlier on weekdays). The change in sleep duration can be a factor, also. A gradual withdrawal from caffeine drinks over a period of several weeks may help alleviate the problem. (Sometimes weekend headaches get worse and are classified as caffeine-withdrawal migraines or rebound headaches — see "Recoiling from Rebound Headaches," later in this chapter.)

The upshot of all this foraging around in Headacheville is this: If your brain's circuitry is sputtering so much that you're spending a lot of time on the sidelines of life, you shouldn't settle for benchwarmer status. Instead, find out what's wrong and what can be done to help. Enlist the aid of your doctor, who brings to the table a wealth of knowledge that can keep you from over-self-medicating and getting discouraged, and can help you arrive at your very own pain solutions.

You may also get a headache because you have dental problems or a sinus infection, or you're withdrawing from drugs or caffeine.

Now that the migraine-busting club is in session, please record the minutes (in your headache journal) — and have the sergeant-at-arms usher out all migraine-triggers, saboteurs, and head-floggers.

Understanding What Makes a Migraine a Migraine

A good starting point is defining what a migraine actually is — an issue that undoubtedly flips through your mind once or twice when you're lying on your bed, grasping your head, wondering what this madness is all about.

First, you need to understand that a migraine isn't just a headache. Oh, no. It's a headache and more — or the more without the headache.

Headaches aren't the only symptom of migraines. Migraines are an umbrella for multiple symptoms, one of which is the headache (and even the headaches come in a wide range of painfulness).

Basically, if you have throbbing head pain along with three (or more) of the symptoms described in Chapter 2, you probably have migraines. Most people have migraines without *auras* (visual disturbances, such as flashing lights, that precede the headache), but some do experience migraines with auras.

Migraine headaches are intermittent — once a week, perhaps, or once a month or year — you don't have them every day. However, a single headache can last for days.

Some migraine symptoms are also indicative of other medical conditions, such as stroke or seizure. So you need to see your doctor to confirm the diagnosis of migraine.

Because everyone's migraines are a bit different, your reality may be some combination of common migraine symptoms, but you can generally expect symptoms similar to the following:

✔ Pain

• Affects one side of the head

• Is moderate to severe to almost unbearable

• Can be described as "throbbing" or "hammering"

• May last two hours to three days or more

✔ Stomach symptoms include

• Lack of appetite

• Stomach pain

• Nausea or vomiting (after which you feel better)

• Constipation and/or diarrhea

✔ Sensory symptoms include

• Sensitivity to light, noise, or smells

• Visual disturbances (zigzagging or flashing lights, or partial vision) that precede your head pain (see auras in Chapter 2)

✔ Symptoms in your limbs include

• Weakness in an arm or leg, or both

• Tingling and/or numbness in your arms and face

• Cold hands and feet

You may also feel disoriented or dizzy, and you may experience mood changes — you feel unusually lethargic and "down."

Keeping the faith

Sometimes it takes a while to realize that the headaches you're experiencing are migraines. One guy looked for help for his horrible migraines for years. He had riveting pain that was "like a jackhammer," and it took two or three days for him to come out of the pain and fog. He went to bed in a darkened room, and his daughter brought him fast-food and drinks until he felt better.

Finally, after living with migraines for 10 years, he went to a headache specialist. The headache specialist got him involved in working up a regimen for pain relief. The prescription medication (a triptan) worked far better than anything he had taken in the past. (For info about medications, see Chapter 8.) He used relaxation techniques and began doing weight-training. Today, although he still has them occasionally, his headaches are less debilitating, and he finally feels like he "has a life."

His biggest regret is that he waited so long to look for genuine solutions. He just tried to grit his teeth and bear the pain. "I thought having migraines was unmanly, so I suffered for years just because of the stigma. I didn't want my doctor to think I was a total wimp."

Tracking the stages of a migraine

Rarely is a migraine as simple as "just the headache pain." Sometimes it *is* just that — no more, no less. Often, though, migraines come with other symptoms (see the previous section). Your symptoms may usher you through some or all of the phases/stages described in the following list:

- **Prodrome:** This stage may occur anytime from a few hours to two days before a headache begins. You may feel an extraordinary sensitivity to lights, sounds, and smells. Your mood may be gloomy or blue, although some people are downright euphoric during this stage. Many people yawn. Your hands and feet may feel cold.

- **Aura:** Some migraine sufferers have this stage, but most don't. The aura usually amounts to a brief period (15 to 45 minutes) of visual disturbances. Less common symptoms include numbness, weakness, or even changes in the way you see things. (See Chapter 2 for more on auras.)

- **Headache:** This phase can last anywhere from two hours to three days (the duration of migraines varies greatly). The Big Kahuna Migraine pitches a tent in your head to stay for a while — this can be painful, nauseating, dizzying, and more. The onset of the pain is usually gradual. The pain may be felt on one or both sides of your head, or it may change sides during your headache.

- **Recovery and postdrome:** The headache finally fades, leaving you in a bummed-out slump during which you feel like you've been drawn and quartered. The postdrome phase typically lasts about a day. During this phase, you may feel physically worthless. On the other hand, some folks in postdrome move into a full-tilt energy phase, totally high on life because they're finally free of the pain. Some even experience a truly euphoric day of huge productivity, much like the mood that is sometimes seen in prodrome.

Figure 4-1 charts the whole process.

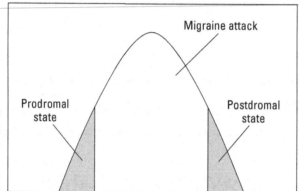

Figure 4-1:
Charting the
course of a
migraine.

Tracing the trek through your brain

Investigators believe that you can blame the symptoms of migraine — from pain to vomiting to aura — on specific brain-related changes. The blood vessels, by the way, are viewed as the supporting actors in the grand drama of the migraine, while the nerve cells appear to be the rabble-rousers.

Well, even if you don't care about the scoop on the birth of a migraine, or you don't think that it makes much sense, all you really need is a general idea of the thrashing-about that's going on in your brain in order to understand why the chaos can make your head hurt.

Researchers think that migraine headaches come from a disturbed blood flow to the brain that results when arteries first narrow and then swell. The *vascular theory* — that a migraine results from the expansion of blood vessels in the brain — is no longer believed. Many migraine-treatment medications that constrict dilated vessels have effects on systems beyond blood circulation.

Scientists had long noted that migraine pain occurred when blood vessels on the surface of the brain dilated, but *why* they dilated was less of an issue. As it turns out, these headaches originate in the brain stem, and the pain arises from changes in brain chemistry. The prevalent belief now is that the migraine-prone person gets exposed to a trigger (or triggers), and then brain cells emit chemicals that cause the expansion of blood vessels on the surface of the brain. The vessels, upon widening, stimulate nerve fibers, thus resulting in throbbing pain.

The head honchos on headaches (the people who do headache research and study scientific evidence) contend that problems with the brain's *neurotransmitters* (brain-messenger chemicals) are the real villains behind migraine and tension-type headaches, which were previously (and erroneously) called muscle-contraction headaches. Communication between the neurotransmitters and brain cells (neurons) breaks down, and the levels of serotonin and other brain-messenger chemicals fluctuate — a big problem for your body, because serotonin plays a role in your ability to feel pain. Therefore, when migraineurs take medications that affect their serotonin levels, many of them get better fast. (See Chapter 8 for medications.)

Migraines are generated in the brain stem. When pain centers of the brain stem get revved up, the spreading excitation appears to stimulate blood vessels and nerves in the brain. Thus, a migraine can occur when a person has a genetic tendency and certain neurochemical changes take place in the brain, leading to a spiral that results in the brain doing quirky chemical cartwheels that spur a vascular process. Why? The chemical brain messengers are thrown off balance, which irritates the blood vessels and thus alters blood flow to the brain. After this occurs, pain signals are sent back to the brain stem.

Getting inside your head for a closer look

Today's high-tech imaging equipment thrills researchers! With help from some very cool imaging equipment, they can get inside the heads of migraine sufferers and actually watch what happens in the brain when a migraine attack occurs.

The ability to view the brain during a migraine attack has helped clarify the migraine mechanism somewhat. Researchers have noted that the brain's neurons are more hyperactive than normal during migraine headaches. And it appears that the activity shoots down from the top of the brain to the brain stem, where key pain centers are found. In people who have migraines (but not other headache types), this rampant electrical feistiness takes place in the brain stem. So some researchers have concluded that

migraine pain either springs from the revving up of these pain centers in the brain stem or from the blood vessels and nerves around the brain getting stimulated from spreading excitation.

The migraine aura is believed to be due to a wave of electrical excitation that moves across the surface of the brain. It is followed by the depression of electrical activity. The electrical activity can activate pain nerves and start the migraine headache.

You have to figure one more fact into the equation: The migraine sufferer must be exposed to triggers (or just one trigger) — a combination of menstrual hormones, a specific type of food, and high anxiety, for example — that set the fright-night headache in motion.

Identifying Variations on the Migraine Theme

As if migraines aren't big enough mischief-makers as it is, they also like to sing show tunes and take on different personas. So here we turn to *migraine variants* — the exceptions and odd lots that make finding your way to migraine diagnosis and treatment quite a challenging proposition.

Abdominal migraines

Abdominal migraines, which are sometimes diagnosed in children, are unusual because they cause pain in the stomach and lead to nausea and vomiting (sometimes without a headache).

A child who complains of recurrent pain in his stomach may be experiencing abdominal migraines. Children who suffer from abdominal migraines are likely to have migraine headaches in adulthood. Abdominal migraines are usually treated with anticonvulsant drugs. (See Chapter 20 for more on abdominal migraines in children.)

Basilar migraines

The basilar migraine was once known as the basilar artery migraine, or BAM. It was considered to be a problem that was found primarily in young women and adolescent girls, but it occurs in both sexes and all ages. Basilar migraines are extremely rare, but they have the potential to be a serious health hazard in that they can lead to a transient ischemic attack (TIA) or stroke.

Symptoms to watch for are double vision, partial vision loss, terrible vomiting, dizziness, loss of balance, slurred speech, lack of coordination, numbness (on one or both sides of the body), weakness, and confusion. These symptoms typically go away at the onset of the actual headache, although they may last for days after the pain disappears.

If you experience any of the symptoms that signal basilar migraines, see a doctor as soon as possible.

Transient ischemic attacks, which can result from basilar migraines (although they rarely do), are essentially "mini-strokes." TIAs result from disruptions of the blood flow to the brain. Although a stroke can mean permanent disability, TIAs don't cause lasting damage. Any neurologic problems associated with TIAs, such as weakness in one arm and slurred speech, are resolved within 24 hours.

Hemiplegic migraines

Hemiplegic migraines are often caused by an inherited gene, but they occur in people with no family history of migraines. With hemiplegic migraines, you experience temporary paralysis or arm and leg weakness on one side of your body. The paralysis or weakness is then followed, usually within an hour, by bad head pain. The paralysis or weakness does not always go away when the headache disappears. These headaches often originate during childhood.

Ocular migraines

Ocular migraines are rare migraines that feature a repeated vision distur- bance (temporary, partial, or complete vision loss in one eye) that lasts less than one hour. After the vision disturbance subsides, you're left with a dull ache behind the affected eye, and your entire head may ache, as well.

If you suffer from ocular migraines, you need to be evaluated by a doctor (an ophthalmologist) to exclude other possible causes for your vision loss.

Ophthalmoplegic migraines

Ophthalmoplegic migraines are no longer believed to be migraines. They are now thought to be a type of *neuritis* (inflammation of a nerve). These headaches are associated with pain around the eyeball and the temporary weakness or paralysis of eye muscle(s). It's a condition that's usually diag- nosed in children. The common symptoms of these migraines are a drooping eyelid, a dilated pupil, and double vision.

Ophthalmoplegic migraines, which can last for days or months, require a thorough exam and testing to rule out conditions that are more serious.

Status migrainosus

The term *status migrainosus* refers to a migraine attack that goes on for more than 72 hours and leads to problems such as dehydration.

If you have status migrainosus, you should go to the emergency room, where you will be treated with IV fluids and pain medication.

Women-only migraines

Certain migraines are uniquely attached to the hormonal swings that females experience. Migraines are commonly linked to menstruation. Some women get migraine headaches when they're on oral contraceptives. And in the case of women who are going through or are past menopause, hormone therapy migraines can be problematic. (Some older women have hormone-replacement-therapy-related headaches, while other women who have had migraines in the past no longer have them after menopause.) See Chapter 19 for more on women and migraines.

Recoiling from Rebound Headaches

A *rebound headache* is a headache that you end up with just because you go in search of a little relief from the constant pounding in your noggin. You feel bad, so you take a pill — you feel worse, so you take another, and so on, and so on, and scoobie-doobie-do. Basically, you wind up with a headache because you're overusing medications.

Exceeding label or physician instructions when taking medications can result in rebounding into another headache. Other spin-offs of medication overuse include a more excruciatingly painful headache, addiction to medications, and other adverse side effects. Prolonged use of even over-the-counter medicines can cause liver and kidney damage.

In the wild-and-woolly migraine arena, rebound headaches have to rank right up there at the top of the pain-wielding, mind-blowing, frustration-inciting extravaganza. Sometimes rebound headaches are migraines, and sometimes they're not.

To help prevent future rebound headaches, you may be able to take a migraine-preventive medication or use lifestyle changes without medication. First, however, you must get past the vicious cycle of rebounding — you overmedicate over and over before realizing that you're perpetuating your pain. Your doctor can help you taper off your overmedicating, nonproductive ways.

If some of the following signs apply to you, you're probably having rebound headaches (but be sure to see your doctor for evaluation of your problem to confirm that it's a headache and not something more serious):

✔ You suffer from headaches daily or every other day.

✔ Your pain intensifies about three hours after your last dose of medication.

✔ Your pain medications don't work as well as they used to.

✔ You take more medication, but your headaches are worse.

✔ You rely on more pills, and you take them more often.

✔ You take medication even for mild headaches, and you often try to ward off a headache by using a medication.

✔ You take pain relievers three to four days a week, and you average more than three tablets per day. (This depends on the kind of medication you're taking, so you'll need your doctor's advice.)

✔ Your pain runs the gamut from mild to moderate to horrible. Usually, the pain is a dull ache that you feel on both sides of your forehead and, sometimes, on the top or back of your head.

✔ Your headaches occur much more frequently.

Because you're in pain, you may use medications too often. The theory behind the rebound headache is that the overuse of drugs makes the headache rebound after your body has absorbed all of the medication. Painkillers are supposed to relieve pain, of course, but if you overuse prescription or nonprescription drugs, they can turn on you and actually cause headaches.

Essentially, an over-the-counter drug or a prescription medication that's taken too often can give rise to a brain-craving for more of the medicine. The episode begins when the brain gets some initial relief from pain, likes the effect, and then decides it will send out to room service for more of the same. Your brain continues to signal "pain" in its search for more of the drug, and you have to take increasing dosages to get relief. Therefore, your medication becomes less and less effective, and you create a cycle of increasing misery.

If you rush to the emergency room with a killer migraine, the doctor will want to know what you took and when you took it last, so be prepared to supply this information. The emergency room physician needs to know if you overused medication and have a rebound headache. She doesn't want to treat you with a medication you overused, or with a medication that's not going to jibe with a drug you took recently.

The typical medications that appear in the rebound scenario are aspirin and acetaminophen, alone or in combination with caffeine-containing products. Other drug culprits often implicated in rebounding are

✔ Caffeine

✔ Codeine

✔ Combination drugs such as Fiorinal and Midrin

✔ Drugs containing barbiturates

✔ Ergotamine tartrate

✔ Opiates

Abortive drugs (such as the nonsteroidals ibuprofen and naproxen), triptans (Imitrex, Zomig, Amerge), and DHE (dihydroergotamine) may also induce rebounding, but they're less likely to do so.

For more details about medications, see Chapters 7 and 8.

Knowing what can make you feel worse

Rebound headaches occur innocently enough: You feel a headache coming on, so you take an over-the-counter pain reliever, such as ibuprofen, aspirin, or acetaminophen, or a prescription medication, such as the oft-prescribed Midrin. Ordinarily, the drug you take works well, and you use it on an occasional basis. This time, however, you don't get relief soon enough. So you take the daily recommended dose (or more) three times during one week, and the result is a rebound headache that's worse and longer-lasting than the one you had to begin with.

Another route for getting a rebound is trying to stave off a headache — because you remember how painful your last migraine was, you begin taking medication at the first hint of a headache.

Too many meds

As a rule, you risk a rebound headache if you take pain relievers for more than two days in a row, in a seven-day period. Depending on the particular medication, taking even one or two pills of a prescription medication per day is enough to result in a rebound headache in many people, but it's more typical for someone to take more than one or two tablets.

The phrase *analgesic rebound headache* refers specifically to the excessive use of pain relievers — a major factor in the transformation of episodic migraine into chronic daily headache, often called *transformed migraine.*

Desperate but dumb

We heard about a guy whose everlasting headache pushed him over the edge of the abyss into a horrible pain place. He thought that his migraine was going to last forever. He had it for six days, and he kept taking one medication after another, but nothing helped.

Finally, he took some pills that his housemate used to help relieve a headache he had after a surgical procedure. After a day of dosing with his housemate's pills, he was suspended in a terrible headache. Feeling very panicky, he called his doctor, who had him stop taking both kinds of medications and try some ways to get pain relief without drugs. After two days of relaxation techniques and head massages, he finally rejoined the land of the living.

A few too many OTC drugs — and, ay, carumba! What a headache!

We know a New York–based flight attendant who was taking OTC drugs to self treat her headaches. She had not been diagnosed with migraines, but she thought that her headaches resembled the migraines her mother had always experienced.

"Everybody's taking something for headaches, and I was definitely gulping a lot of pills. Finally, as it turned out, my episodic headaches were transformed into chronic daily headaches, or that's how the ER doctor explained it when my fiancé took me to the emergency room. I was lying down in the car and my head was splitting — I really, truly thought I was dying. The doctor had me see a headache specialist,

who told me I'd had a rebound or drug-induced headache. He said that both over-the-counter and prescription meds can cause rebounding if they're taken too often."

Looking back, she is glad that her "crisis" led her to get help — something she should have done years earlier. "My doctor told me that I wouldn't have gotten better on my own, and that rebounding can be very painful and troublesome. He took me off these drugs, and it was two months before I finally quit having frequent headaches. Then, he helped me come up with a treatment plan that was much healthier and targeted my migraines better."

An analgesic is basically a pain-relief medication. Non-narcotic analgesics such as acetaminophen (Tylenol) are used to treat mild- to medium-pain migraines. Some analgesic products contain caffeine as an added ingredient to help pump up the pain-killing impact.

Overusing OTC medications that contain caffeine often leads to rebound headaches. Consider the fact that some of these tablets contain up to 60 mg of caffeine per pill. Therefore, if you take 10 tablets a day — not extraordinary for a migraine sufferer — you get quite a major pile-up of caffeine.

Too much or too little caffeine

Adding to the risk of rebound headaches is excessive caffeine consumption. If you drink four or more cups of coffee (or six colas or cups of tea) a day, you may have trouble.

You may also get rebound headaches or weekend migraines when you fail to consume your usual amount of caffeine. If you normally drink seven cups of coffee at work, Monday through Friday, and then you drop down to one cup on Saturday, the drastic plummet in caffeine intake can give your body a jolt. The drop in caffeine may cause your blood vessels to widen and lead to a migraine. This example drives home a fact that many migraine sufferers have discovered the hard way — you can't drink five cups of coffee and other caffeinated drinks per day and then suddenly just cut yourself off, unless you want to suffer a mammoth headache.

To cut back on your intake of caffeine, use a tapering-off approach. Start by cutting down slightly on coffee, cola, chocolate, and tea, and keep reducing your consumption by 6 ounces each week. Also, reduce your use of caffeine-containing medication. To avoid a withdrawal headache, stay at each new intake level for several days. If possible, set your sights on a caffeine-free diet, which is ideal for your overall health and your avoidance of migraines.

Getting off the rebound treadmill

What's the answer for rebound headaches? Stop taking the medications that are causing you trouble. In the case of nonprescription drugs, stop taking them immediately, or taper off over two to three days.

If you have questions about how to taper off your offending medication, or if you're still hurting from the vicious circle-pain-rebound migraine, call your doctor for advice. Your doctor may start you on a preventive medication, but it won't be very effective until you discontinue using the overused medication and it's out of your system. (The length of time that drugs stay in your system varies greatly, depending on the drug, so you need to rely on your doctor's advice when discontinuing the use of a drug.)

During your withdrawal from the offending medication(s), which can take several weeks, your headaches get worse before they get better. Within a few hours after you stop taking the drugs, your head begins to hurt even more, and the pain continues to gain momentum for a day or two. Have your doctor monitor your progress and, if necessary, give you a transition dose of a medication that you can use temporarily to get past the rough spots.

Hospitalization may be necessary if you're discontinuing the long-term use of ergotamine or narcotics (opiates). You must detox from these medications to reduce migraine frequency and free up your system to be responsive to preventives.

Naturally, you may feel oh so stupid and silly for perpetuating your own headache by taking too many pills, but don't think that it's just you — most migraine sufferers do this at some point. When you're caught in a pain trap and you can't get out, you try almost anything — and that's how you got on the rebound merry-go-round in the first place. Just make a point of etching firmly in your mind how very awful a rebound headache can be. This thought will slap down your hand the next time you're a bit hasty in reaching for your pain medications.

This cycle of dependency is both frightening and hard to handle. Sometimes the only solution is to slap an ice pack or cooling pad on your head and ride it out cold turkey. (Repeat a positive affirmation: "This will spiral to an end at some point. Within 24 hours — this time tomorrow — the pain will be gone.")

Biofeedback and behavioral therapy are sometimes used to treat mood disturbances that are occasionally associated with chronic daily headaches (see Chapter 9).

Typically, people who work on reducing their dependency to medications after experiencing the rebound crucible eventually reach a plateau where they have migraines less often, and the migraines aren't as bad as previous ones. In most cases of rebound, the long-term outcome is very promising. Moreover, you don't have to fear another rebound skirmish, because your doctor can provide you with an improved treatment plan for future migraines.

Defusing the Myths

Migraines often go undiagnosed for years. Many people flounder around with the pain and other symptoms and fail to get proper solutions because they're trapped in the migraine myths, such as "what you have isn't a migraine, because my brother has them, and he always throws up, and you don't" or "people who have migraines are always depressed."

No, she wasn't going crazy

No, you're not imagining things or trying to creep people out when you say that your head hurts like crazy. So will someone please listen?

Sometimes it's super-difficult to get headaches diagnosed correctly. You may feel a little goony just having them, and you really hate getting into all the gruesome details. Or you're afraid that when you try to bring up the subject, your doctor will think that you're some whining little hypochondriac, or that you're wildly exaggerating. Sound familiar?

A Houston postal worker had headaches so debilitating that she was missing work often. The situation scared her because, as a single mom, she was the only wage-earner in the family, and it was her job to "bring home the bacon and fry it up in a pain." What if she got fired for missing so much work?

Soft-spoken and undemanding, this woman mentioned her headaches to her gynecologist, who patted her hand and told her that she was under a lot of stress as a single mother. He didn't ask about other symptoms, and she didn't volunteer any information. But the truth was, bright lights made her headaches worse, and over-the-counter meds never helped. Plus, she felt nauseated every time a headache hit, which was invariably right around the time she began her period each month.

One day, she casually unloaded her symptoms on a customer who was writing a book on migraines (and buying stamps). The writer told her that the symptoms sounded like migraine. But she said, "No, my doctor didn't diagnose me with migraines."

There's the rub. Who knows more about your own hurting head than you? Try to convey all of your symptoms to your doctor, because one thing is for sure — he won't be able to guess them!

Despite myths to the contrary, migraines are real and valid physical problems that require concrete solutions. Your migraine probably carries a whole constellation of sidekick symptoms that need to be addressed. In other words, pulling yourself up by your bootstraps just won't do it. (For more on handling the responses of others, see Chapters 16 and 17.) Don't let anyone tell you that the pain is "all in your head." It's not! Hard-throbbing head pain is certainly not the stuff fantasies are made of.

Some folks think that they know exactly what constitutes a migraine; other folks only know what migraines aren't. Table 4-1 lays out some of the common myths and realities of migraines.

Table 4-1	Migraine Myths and Realities
Myth	**Reality**
Migraines have certain, specific symptoms that make them migraines, and if your headaches are at all different, they're not migraines.	There are a multitude of migraine symptoms, of which one symptom or a combination of symptoms indicates a true migraine.
All migraineurs have the same symptoms.	Migraineurs experience different symptoms. Migraines are very individualistic. Your migraines may be totally different from those of another migraine sufferer you happen to know.
Migraines are psychological, not physiological.	Migraines are definitely physiological in nature, causing distinct neurological changes. They're not just "in your head."
Your doctor is completely familiar with all migraine symptoms and should be able to diagnose you just by hearing that you have headaches sometimes.	Some doctors are more adept at headache diagnosis than others. But even the most skilled diagnostician will need you to provide a clear picture of your headaches to aid him in diagnosing your head pain.

If you want your physician to have your treasure-trove of personal health history at his fingertips, you must be good at info-sharing. So if you tell your family doctor that you have occasional headaches that are killers, but you fail to flesh the symptoms out, your physician won't have enough information to help you. Be as specific as possible. See Chapters 5 and 6 for guidelines on making sure that your headaches are diagnosed correctly.

You have to be your number-one advocate in healthcare delivery. You should know your body better than anyone else; you should be quite familiar with your existing health conditions and the medications you take. You're definitely a pro at describing what's troubling you. Your valuable input allows you and your physician to cut through myths and misconceptions and get to the truth.

Chapter 5

Finding a Good Migraine Doctor

. . . .

In This Chapter

▶ Seeing your healthcare provider

▶ Is your doctor migraine-friendly?

▶ Moving on to a specialist, if necessary

▶ Prepping for the migraine specialist

. . . .

Doctor, doctor, give me the news! Even if you're virtually clueless about your headaches' why, when, where, and pretty much everything else, don't let it keep you from seeking medical help. You start with the basics, but you ultimately want to end up with a physician who knows the latest and greatest treatments and is sensitive to your problem.

Seeing Your Everyday Doc

You're sick of hurting, and you figure that you've been a stoical person for long enough. Time to take this problem to the doctor! (By the way, you can rest assured that getting help is a terrific idea, because, contrary to what you may have heard, there's a lot you can do to help alleviate your headaches. The "grin and bear it" thing is so over.)

If you're not getting pain relief from over-the-counter (OTC) headache remedies, set up an appointment to see your primary care doctor. For this very important under-the-hood inspection, you can start with your primary care doctor and see if she can key in on your headache type successfully.

However, if your headaches prove to be more than a little perplexing, and your healthcare provider is conflicted in her opinion on what kind you have, go on to the next level — a headache specialist, who probably spends a large percentage of her time focusing on headache diagnosis and treatment. (See Chapter 6.)

Knowing when to go

See your doctor if any one of the following conditions describes your headache situation:

- ✔ You get headaches as frequently as once a month.

- ✔ Sometimes you feel so bad, that you can't go to work.

- ✔ Your headaches last for hours or days.

- ✔ Over-the-counter drugs rarely provide relief.

- ✔ You're 50 (or older) and you just started having headaches.

- ✔ Your headaches have changed — they're getting more severe, or they occur more often than in the past.

- ✔ You experience other symptoms along with your headaches, such as vision problems, hallucinations, balance troubles, light sensitivity, and so on.

- ✔ You get headaches after various kinds of exertion (from aerobics to straining during difficult bowel movements).

If you have any of the symptoms listed as danger signs in Chapter 18 and on the Cheat Sheet at the front of this book, go straight to the emergency room. (In some rare instances, a headache can be extremely serious.)

Previewing the procedure

What happens when you visit your doctor? You describe your headaches and symptoms. Or you can give your doctor your handy headache journal (see Chapter 3). If you haven't had time to fill out a headache journal, be ready to describe your headache's frequency and severity, as well as any triggers you suspect. Also, be sure to provide your medical history and specifics on any medications you're taking (for head pain and otherwise).

Your mission is to get your physician up to speed on your headache story: frequency, duration, how disabling the headaches are, and possible triggers.

You also need to let your doctor know what you used to try to make the pain go away: the cooling pads you put on your aching head, the types of medications you took (that didn't help), or the pretending-that-it's-not-really-happening denial thing.

To help with the diagnosis, your doctor may ask you to fill out a form called a Migraine Disability Assessment Scale (MIDAS) or a Headache Impact Test (HIT), or your doc may just ask you questions. A headache specialist will want the answers to the following questions:

✔ What's the timing and length of your headaches?

- What time of day do you get them?

- Do your headaches come and go within the same day or the same week?

- What time of the month do you get them? (Before or during your period, for example.)

- How long does a headache usually last?

✔ What is your pain like?

- Where do you feel pain — on one side of your head, on both sides of your head, behind one eye, on the front of your head?

- How does the pain feel — like a dull ache, a throbbing pain, mild or excruciating?

- Does the pain move from one spot to another?

- Does the pain creep up and get worse, or does it slam you suddenly?

✔ What other symptoms do you get with your headaches?

- Do you feel nauseated?

- Do you vomit?

✔ What do you use to try to alleviate your headaches?

- What medications or solutions have you tried, and did these provide any relief?

- Do you take any vitamin supplements or herbal supplements?

- What are your headache triggers?

- Do you get a headache from skipping meals?

- Do you get a headache after eating certain foods?

- Do your headaches follow physical activity, such as sex or exercise?

- Have you noticed a connection between extreme stress and the start of a headache?

✔ What factors may have contributed to your having headaches?

- Have you had any kind of head trauma, such as from a car accident or sports injury?

- Do others in your family have headaches?

✔ When did you first start having headaches?

✔ Have you noticed anything that seems to make the pain worse when you have a headache?

The info you provide and the examination your doctor performs point the way toward the best methods for headache relief.

Talking about tests you may need

During a typical headache visit, a doctor examines you and asks the questions listed in the previous section. Then she starts eliminating a long list of possibilities. This process is what physicians refer to as a *diagnosis of exclusion.* Using your health information and your description of headaches, your doctor can sort and label: "Okay, it can't be cluster headaches, it's sure not a headache associated with disease, and it's not the stilettos you wear. . ."

Essentially, a headache is diagnosed by evaluating and understanding your medical and headache history and examining you physically. In fact, your doctor may diagnose your headache without doing a single test.

No blood test or imaging method can diagnose the common types of headache. Tests generally aren't necessary unless your doctor isn't able to arrive at a diagnosis and wants to check for other, more unusual causes. (See Chapter 6 for more on tests.)

The wonderful news is this: Most patients who seek help in finding a treatment plan for their headaches do get pain relief.

Asking about short-term precautions

You and your doctor may have to work your way through trial-and-error before you're able to zero in on the best approach for treating your headaches.

No matter what the outcome of your doctor visit, be sure to ask your doctor what short-term precautions you should take to help alleviate your headaches, as well as how you can avoid sabotaging yourself. Your doctor will probably want you to follow these guidelines:

- ✔ Don't smoke.

- ✔ Get plenty of rest, and try to sleep about the same number of hours per night.

- ✔ Be on the lookout for possible headache triggers — foods, smells, sounds, lights — that set a headache into motion.

- ✔ If you drink coffee, try to cut down your consumption gradually. When you get down to one cup in the morning (for example), drink it at about the same time each day.

Caffeine can trigger migraines, but withdrawal can also cause awful headaches.

✔ Low-key exercise can make you healthier and, therefore, help you stave off headaches. Walk a mile or so, three or four times a week. Start gradually and only do what you can handle.

✔ Don't exceed dose recommendations on over-the-counter headache remedies, and don't exceed your doctor's instructions for prescription drugs.

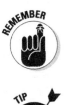

Often, people who suffer from migraines get desperate to eliminate the pain (or they may get confused about how many tablets they've taken) and take more pills in a day than they should. The result can be a rebound headache, which is sometimes so vicious that it makes other headaches absolutely pale in comparison. (See Chapter 4 for more on rebound headaches.)

If your doctor suggests a headache plan, ask her how long it will take for the approach to provide relief.

Discovering Whether Your Physician Understands Migraines

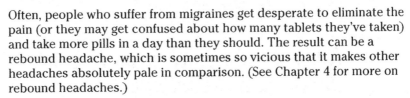

So you go to see your doctor, and — oops! — you discover that she's just not "into" headache diagnosis. If you're not happy with her response to your concerns, shop around for another doctor. Find a doctor who'll agree to team up with you on a treatment plan. Some primary care doctors are old hands at treating headaches, while others may want to refer you to a headache specialist for diagnosis and treatment. You can also check out doctors on your own.

If your doctor smirks or rolls her eyes when you describe your headache problem, you know you're in trouble. The signals probably won't be that obvious though. So you have to look for subtle clues that let you know that diagnosing and treating headaches just isn't your doc's cup of tea. (You give her a nice case of strep throat, and she's totally in the groove — but headaches aren't her bag.)

Truth is, some doctors aren't very knowledgeable about headache diagnosis and treatment, while others just think in terms of "too many headaches, too little time." Doctors often prefer that you get help from a specialist in the head-pain field — a neurologist, pain-management expert, or internist who has made treating headaches her special passion. However, physicians who don't treat headaches themselves can usually recommend a doctor who specializes in headache diagnosis and treatment. (This specialized doctor's home base may be a headache clinic.)

To determine your doctor's knowledge and interest level, ask some of the questions listed in the section "Screening potential doctors," later in this chapter.

The first doctor you visit may recommend a treatment plan that actually works. But if it doesn't help — or you're worried that you may have a complex problem that requires a specialist — ask your primary care doctor for a referral to a specialist. Don't be shy. Just ask your doctor if she thinks that you should see a headache specialist.

Keeping the faith even if your doctor is a disbeliever

Okay, you weren't thrilled with what your doctor said. You got a pat on the arm and were instructed to "take some acetaminophen," even though you clearly explained that you tried that approach already. If your doctor is skeptical about your headaches, find a headache specialist to diagnose and treat you.

Don't let your doctor's lack of interest keep you from looking further for relief for your headaches. You're definitely doing the right thing by seeking additional opinions. You shouldn't feel any more reluctant to seek help for your headaches than you would if you had a gaping wound or chest pains.

If you feel like you need to see another doctor, or if your doctor refers you to a specialist, don't take it as a sign that you have an awful disease lurking inside you. Actually, the chances of you having a serious health problem is fairly unlikely. You may have high blood pressure, which definitely requires monitoring and medication, or you may just need the right migraine medication and some lifestyle changes (see Chapter 8 for more on medications, and the chapters in Part IV for lifestyle suggestions).

Giving up on finding help is a really bad idea. Help is out there, it just may take a little effort to find it.

Spotting signs that you need to look elsewhere for a doctor

What do you do if your doctor seems marginal about treating headaches? She wants to help you, but she doesn't appear to be overflowing with headache knowledge. Or she is clearly leaning toward sending you to someone whom she considers better equipped to diagnose your problem.

You need to be able to identify the components of a deal-breaker, the indications that point you to the exit door so that you can do some more doctor shopping. If you notice even one of these signals, keep looking for a doctor to treat your headaches:

- Your doctor makes a dismissive comment: "Well, after all, this is just a headache — not exactly anything earthshaking. . . ." or "Women have a lot of headaches due to hormone changes. . . ."

- Your doctor looks bored when you describe your symptoms, as if she has heard all this a million times before.

- Your doctor seems eager to refer you to a specialist.

- Your doctor looks confused when you describe your headache symptoms.

- Your doctor comes from the bite-the-bullet treatment school and wants you to go to bed and tough it out until the headache goes away (obviously, this healthcare provider has never had migraines herself).

- Your doctor doesn't discuss your medical history or answer your questions. (We refer to doctors who are treating migraines, but be advised that this is not a good sign of a helpful healthcare provider in any domain!)

- Your physician seems eager to finish up and suggests a pain medication right away.

- Your diagnosis is still up in the air after a visit or two.

You may want to shop around for a headache specialist if your primary care physician tells you that she doesn't feel comfortable trying to diagnose and treat your severe headaches, or if an existing medical problem leads you to believe that you may benefit from seeing a headache specialist. You may also need a headache specialist if you take over-the-counter medications almost every day, and you don't get any new solutions when you visit your doctor.

 If you see disinterest or reluctance on the part of your doctor to work with you on migraine management, don't hesitate to ask for a referral to a headache specialist. The specialist will probably be a neurologist or internist who specializes in treating migraines.

Turning to a Headache Specialist

So, you're moving on to a headache specialist. This step makes sense for most migraineurs — everyone except those lucky enough to have their regular doctor be a headache guru.

Even if you're in an HMO, you can switch doctors and get another opinion. You have to call your insurance company and make an official change of your PCP (primary care provider). The new doctor must be on your insurance company's list. If the new doctor is not on your insurance company's list, you'll have to pay all fees out-of-pocket (your pocket).

Finding a competent migraine specialist

Finding the right healthcare provider to diagnose and treat your headaches can be tricky. Aunt Ethel swears by her chiropractor, and officemate Kara Lynn has used a neurologist.

Perhaps you already saw one specialist, and to you, a pain-management guy sounds like the best diagnostician and treatment-dispenser. Then again, you once dated someone who found headache relief from an acupuncturist, and you wonder if you should check out that option. (The date was a bust, but you liked the headache tale.)

Depending on the suspected cause of your headaches, your primary care doctor may advise you to see a neurologist, allergist, ophthalmologist, or ear, nose, and throat doctor. Treatment will vary depending on the problem behind your headaches.

- Neurologists are especially well-qualified to diagnose headaches because their specialty is the central nervous system, the key area that gives rise to migraines.

- Allergists may be helpful if your primary care physician suspects that allergies are behind your headaches.

- Ophthalmologists (a doctor who treats the eye) are a good option if your primary care doctor believes that your headaches may be related to eye problems.

- Internists may be good doctors for headache diagnosis because they have a wide range of medical knowledge. (Some specialize in headache diagnosis, in particular.)

- Ear, nose, and throat doctors can treat headaches associated with such conditions as chronic sinus infections.

Don't choose your healthcare provider on the basis of a large and glitzy ad in a health magazine or because she's located next to a great spa where you can get a massage and body wrap after your doctor appointment. A large, impressive advertisement or a clinic in a good location has little to do with the doctor's credentials and experience in diagnosing and treating headaches. Therefore, you can't consider these characteristics to be a sign of her potential success in handling your head-pain problem.

One caveat: Use a fringe specialist (acupuncturist, chiropractor, and so on) only after you've been evaluated by at least a primary care doctor and a serious cause of your headaches has been excluded — and if someone at your local medical center offers resounding testimonials for the specialist's headache-treating skills. Not having a medical-school background is a drawback when you're dealing with an issue as complicated as headaches.

The hunt for a competent migraine specialist may take a month or so, but hopefully this represents a very small slice of the long life stretched out in front of you — an existence that will be far better lived with less pain from headaches. The trick is finding a healthcare provider to help you lasso those migraines, get them under control, and tie them up in the old corral.

Getting referrals

A good way to find someone to treat your headaches is to use the same approach you'd take if you were looking for an expert in any field — a great hairstylist or someone to remove a bunion, for example. Ask around, and check references, credentials, and resources. Exhaust your networking circle.

Gather information from family and friends, but keep your mind set on being a good consumer. Your mom may say, "I like to go to Sunrise Clinic because it's only a mile from my house — I can walk to it!" This reasoning may be absolutely okay if you're choosing a post office or restaurant, but not if you're looking for someone to treat your head pain!

Treat your selection of a doctor as a major decision. Make sure that you use considerable caution when scrutinizing all the input you're given.

List a few of the doctors that your friends and family recommend, and check out their credentials. You want a doctor who regularly treats headaches, has a good reputation, and is respected by other doctors. Your primary care doctor is a good source for finding a headache specialist.

Checking with medical centers and universities

You can call the National Headache Foundation, your city's medical association, or your state's medical association to get some names of doctors who can diagnose and treat your headaches. Then you can look for the names on your health insurance carrier's list of doctors if you want to make sure that the fees are at least partially covered by your insurance. You can ask your primary care doctor for a recommendation on a headache specialist.

Did I see you yawning?

You have every right to expect your doctor to take your headaches seriously. A woman we know was dismayed when her gynecologist's eyes glazed over after she told him how awful her migraines were. "I could tell he thought, 'Oh, no, not another woman whining about headaches!' It made me feel stupid, so I shut up. Later, though, when I got home and thought about it, I knew I needed help even if he wasn't the one who could give it to me." She laughs. "The only thing my doctor had told me was 'try to reduce your stress,' and with four children, a bad marriage, and a high-stress job, I knew that wasn't going to happen."

She had such bad headaches that she was missing work at least one day every other week. She couldn't tell if she'd be able to go to her kids' activities, which made it hard to plan for transportation.

"The final straw was missing my daughter's high school graduation — she was one of the top 20 honor students, and I didn't get to see her draped in the gold cords for her achievement. I was stuck in bed at home. I was vomiting and miserable and so sad, because I knew she felt let down. It made me realize I shouldn't have put up with years of telling my problem to the same doctor who was obviously not 'into' headache treatment. I had to take my troubles elsewhere."

She called a local teaching hospital and asked for the names of doctors who were headache specialists. "They gave me two doctor recommendations. I interviewed both of them, and went with the one I felt more comfortable with."

She was diagnosed the first day she met with her doctor. She had migraines, just as she had suspected. "But it took a month to find the best way to combat my headaches. He tried three medications before we found one that worked, and he got me to start a walking program. Now I'm having milder headaches — they're still bothers, but at least I'm able to get out and do things. The abortive drug he prescribed often knocks them out before they get started. I have a much better life now that I finally discovered some solutions. I'd really almost given up on having a good life."

Call a local medical center or university and ask to talk to someone who can give you a doctor referral. Then, pose this key question: "Can you give me the names of three doctors who are headache specialists in this area?"

A local teaching hospital can give you some names of good doctors, and so can your city's medical society or the state medical association. (Check for your state's medical association on the Internet or in the yellow pages of your phone book.)

Two other good referral sources are the American Headache Society (AHS) and the National Headache Foundation. You can contact both of these groups and ask for lists of AHS and NHF members in your state. To reach the National Headache Foundation, you can visit their Web site at www.headaches.org or call 1-888-NHF-5552. To contact the American Headache Society, you can visit their Web site at www.ahsnet.org or call 856-423-0043.

Screening potential doctors

Screening a headache specialist is the easy part. Look for someone with good credentials who has chosen headache diagnosis/treatment as a special area of interest. Find out if the physician treats people for headaches on a daily basis, and ask how many years of experience she has. But don't rule out a promising young doctor (who has only a few years of experience) if you're otherwise impressed with her, or an internist who is good at treating headaches even though it's only one part of her practice.

The following questions will help you determine if you've found a knowledge-able headache physician.

- ✔ How long have you been treating headaches?

- ✔ How often do you treat people who have headaches?

- ✔ Are you board-certified (or board-eligible) in your specialty? (In the United States and Canada, doctors must pass a board exam to become board-certified, so having this certification means that the doctor has amassed the amount of knowledge required to pass the test.)

- ✔ What are your credentials? Are you a member of any professional headache organizations, such as the National Headache Foundation?

- ✔ Do you take Continuing Medical Education courses to keep yourself abreast of new developments in the diagnosis and treatment of headaches?

- ✔ Have you written or published scientific papers on headaches?

Looking for help in all the right places

We met a headache sufferer who had trouble finding help. "After I described my problem to my gynecologist, he told me I needed a headache specialist. I asked him what the symptoms sounded like to him, and he said his guess was tension but he was 'no expert' on headaches."

So her doctor referred her to a headache specialist, who provided help in a single visit. "The doctor keyed in to what was going on right away — I had food triggers and caffeine withdrawal and about 60 other things that led to migraines, so together we drew up a plan for lifestyle changes, and he prescribed a triptan drug for me to take when I could tell that a headache was first beginning."

The upshot? "I was able to ward off most bad headaches, so I went from having migraines about once a week to once a month. My friends were impressed — they used to come to my apartment and find me either crashed out in bed with a cool pack on my head, vomiting in the bathroom, or throwing goldfish crackers out my window as a distraction from my pain. Now I'm so normal they think I'm boring!"

Before you go to see the doctor, confirm that she works with your insurance company.

Preparing for the Headache Specialist

When you find a doctor that you think can help with your migraines, schedule an appointment right away — and don't wait until you have a headache. You're going to the doctor to develop a plan for managing your headaches, not just to get rid of a headache.

In the doctor's office, don't be afraid to ask the first nurse you meet a few questions about the physician. If anyone seems evasive — or if you get the feeling that there's friction in the office — it's not a good sign. Secret agendas and turmoil in a medical setting won't make for a good (or pleasant) treatment situation. (If you're seeing an alternative-type practitioner, seek a reference from a hospital source in advance.)

When you check in, ask the front office staff the following questions:

- ✔ Does your office help process insurance claims?
- ✔ How far in advance do I need to make an appointment?
- ✔ Do you schedule several patients for the same time slot?
- ✔ How long will I typically wait to see the doctor?

Your doctor will take a medical history to get up-to-date information on your existing medical problems (asthma, diabetes, cancer, and so on) and your headaches. Remember to bring your personal health information, your migraine journal, and any medications you're taking.

If you saw another doctor for your headaches, ask her secretary or nurse to transfer your records. (They will have you sign a medical records release form.) The records can help prevent a duplication of efforts. If you just had an MRI (magnetic resonance imaging) two weeks ago, you don't need another one now.

The headache specialist will examine you and perform a neurological exam that involves checking your reflexes, coordination, and so on. She may also take some lab samples, such as urine and blood.

If you come from a family of migraine sufferers, and your symptoms clearly point to migraine, your doctor may put all your health information together and immediately come up with a diagnosis of migraine. But if the whole thing still looks hazy to the doctor, she'll probably order some tests to help her make a diagnosis. (See Chapter 6 for more information on tests.)

Here are some good queries (along with some acceptable answers) to ask your doctor when she says, "Do you have any questions?"

✔ How do you stay current on the latest headache studies and treatments?

The doctor should read medical journals and keep up to date via continuing education medical courses.

✔ What do you consider when you devise a treatment plan?

The doctor should consider the type of headache, patient preference, and the individual patient's needs.

✔ Can we prepare a written treatment plan that I can take with me?

The doctor should be happy to prepare a written treatment plan.

✔ Will you give me a prescription drug, if necessary?

The doctor should write you a prescription if he feels that medication is necessary.

✔ When treating headaches, what is your goal for the patient?

The doctor's goal should be to provide pain relief and help you attain a good quality of life.

✔ How do you feel about alternative therapies such as acupuncture?

This depends on patient preference. If using an alternative-type therapy is a priority for you, you want to find a doctor who believes in these avenues as complementary therapies.

✔ After you determine the appropriate medication, can you tell me the approximate cost of the drug you prescribe?

The doctor should be happy to discuss the cost of your prescription.

✔ Are there some lifestyle changes I can make instead of taking a prescription drug?

The doctor may be able to offer some suggestions for lifestyle changes that can replace medication, but it depends on her diagnosis. Some headaches can't be alleviated by lifestyle changes alone.

Your doctor will probably say things during your exchange of information and discussion that will inspire additional questions. Don't be shy about asking these questions.

Don't get discouraged if you feel like you're walking through a maze of twisted corridors when you seek headache solutions. If you find good remedies at the end of your quest, you'll forget all the aggravation of keeping a headache journal, giving your medical history, and searching for the right caregiver.

Chapter 6

Having Your Head Examined and Coming Up with a Plan

*Y*ou're seeing a headache specialist. He needs to know your health situation, so an examination and thorough medical and headache history is step one. You present your list of headache details (the foods, activities, and other triggers that lead to your migraines) and other pertinent info. (You can use the headache journal in Chapter 3 to record these things.)

If early solutions for treating your headaches haven't helped, or if your headache symptoms aren't typical or have changed or worsened, your headache specialist may want to run a test or two to help in making a diagnosis. Then, after the results are weighed into the mix, he'll meet with you and come up with an appropriate treatment plan.

If your insurance coverage presents stumbling blocks, you can take steps to unravel the red tape. We give you some tips and tell you how your doctor's office staff can assist you.

Just look at the testing and treatment-planning as phases of your migraine-busting junket that are well worth the time and effort. The likelihood of finding relief is extremely high. If you persist in finding solutions for your migraines, you'll wind up with very viable ways to combat your headaches and, sometimes, prevent them altogether. Now that's a concept you can get your arms (and head) around!

Huddling with Your Doctor

You may be excited when you meet with your headache specialist for some true event planning. This planning session may very well constitute the home stretch of your race toward pain relief. If you're like most people, you'll find concrete answers and pain-relief solutions soon after consulting a headache expert. On the other hand, a period of trial-and-error may be necessary in order to key in on the specific problem.

But even if your trial-and-error phase lasts longer than a few weeks, you can at least feel as though you're doing something to get closer to your ultimate goal — relief from the misery named "headache."

Providing your medical history

You may be able to minimize the medical-history step if you have your records transferred from another doctor that you consulted about your headaches. You can begin your association with the headache specialist by toting some great headache-diagnosing ammo — your headache and medical history, and the results of any tests that were run.

But if it turns out that you're not able to get your records transferred (no matter what you say or do, the transfer never takes place), you'll need to provide all the particulars of your medical history and headache symptoms *one more time*. (Chapter 5 lists the information you need to provide.) If you're keeping a headache diary, it's time to pull it out and share it with your specialist. (See the headache journal in Chapter 3.)

Giving the lowdown on your pain-pill intake

Sometimes people who have headaches downplay the number of pills they take during a pain cycle. If you're one of these people, it doesn't mean that you're a dishonest person. No, it simply shows how tough (and depressing) it is for you to face the magnitude of your pill intake (especially because the medicine didn't work). You may also be foggy-minded during awful headaches, a state that certainly reduces your ability to remember what and how much you took to manage your pain.

Know when to hold 'em, know when to fold 'em

We know an attorney who never liked to admit that he suffered from headaches. The headaches seemed so lame, and he thought of himself as a "manly man." So he wrestled with his pain for many years (from age 16 to 40), missing work and disappointing his children when the family planned things that often had to be cancelled.

Then a business trip to France changed his mind about seeking help. On the flight home, his headache was triggered by the sound of someone repeatedly shuffling a deck of cards. "That sound hit me like a ton of bricks — that and the closed-in feeling of the plane and dehydration and too many airline peanuts. The combo led to a headache so horrible, I wanted to rush to the ER, but instead, I arrived in Houston, alone and in pain, searching for my car in the airport parking lot at 2 a.m. Barely able to function, the pain was so bad, I drove across town the 30 minutes it took to get home, and that did it — I vowed that the suffering had to end. The next day, I made an appointment to see my doctor."

He saw a primary care doctor, who diagnosed him with migraine headaches. He stopped smoking and cut down on drinking alcohol. He had a migraine medication, but he rarely had to use it, because his lifestyle changes helped him have headaches much less often.

"Looking back, I have to thank the card-shuffling guy on the airplane. He sent me running in agony to get help for my migraines!"

Be very up front with your doctor. Tell him what pills you've taken (along with the amount), and let him know how they worked for you and whether you experienced any side effects. He's not in the business of judging people who self-medicate themselves haphazardly — he just wants to help you get better. Besides, in the world of migraine suffering, the overuse of pain pills is alarmingly common.

If you have any special information that may be helpful — perhaps you frequented the ER numerous times because of migraine pain — be sure to share it with your doctor. Also, don't forget to detail any lifestyle factors that may contribute to your condition, such as smoking, caffeine consumption, irregular sleep patterns, skipping meals, and couch-potato status.

You don't need to feel embarrassed when divulging medication information. When migraineurs get caught in the grip of pain-pandemonium, they're naturally going to thrash around for some (any) route out of the headache crucible. You've been there, done that, and you don't want to go back, right? Most importantly, you need to remember that there can be bad interactions between different medications — this is the number one reason for telling your doctor everything about your pill intake.

Taking the Tests

Before you undergo tests, your headache specialist will brief you on the routine for each one. (If he doesn't offer, ask him.) The briefing gives you an idea of what to expect and pretty much eliminates the fear factor. Think of the tests as just another way to get to the bottom of your headache dilemma. These tests may not be very fun, but they help you take a giant step on your road to headache relief.

If you get nervous prior to a test, just tell yourself this comforting old slogan: "This time tomorrow, it will all be over and behind me. I'll be home stretching out in front of the TV and sipping lemonade."

Testing without pencils: Tests you may need

After your headache specialist has absorbed your headache history and personal medical story, he'll do one of two things: tell you what diagnosis he has reached, or brief you on the tests you need to undergo so that he can arrive at a conclusion.

Generally speaking, your doctor will probably want to perform tests if any of the following apply to you:

- ✔ You have bad headaches for the first time.
- ✔ You notice a change in the type of headaches you experience.
- ✔ Your headaches are getting steadily worse.
- ✔ You have neurological symptoms, such as weakness in an arm or leg, or you have an abnormal finding on your eye exam (swollen optic discs).
- ✔ You wake up with a headache.
- ✔ You have headaches after coughing or straining, or after sex or exertion.

At any rate, headaches typically are diagnosed with a physical examination and an overview of the patient's headache and medical history (with no other tests required). Tests generally aren't necessary unless your doctor can't arrive at a clear-cut diagnosis. In this case, he may want to check for other, more unusual or serious causes for your headaches.

If your headaches remain a mystery, your doctor may order a CT scan (see "Tubing your way to a CT scan," later in this chapter), an MRI (see "Making magnetic magic with an MRI," later in this chapter), or a lumbar puncture (see

"Limbering up for a lumbar puncture," later in this chapter). Most of the time, though, a doctor won't need to perform a CT scan, lumbar puncture, or MRI to determine what kind of headaches you're having and how to treat them.

Your doctor may also order some blood tests. These tests can detect many of the medical conditions that sometimes cause headaches — such as infections, thyroid dysfunction, or inflammation of the blood vessels.

The physical examination and the results of the tests will likely show that you don't have an abnormality causing your headache, but the information can enable your doctor to rule out the causes of head pain related to health conditions such as high blood pressure, tumors, and so on.

The purpose of all these tests is to find out what's behind your head pain. They often serve to exclude the more serious causes of headaches — diseases, tumors, and so on. Tests are also sometimes performed to establish a baseline prior to treatment, in other words, to measure where you are now so the medical folk have something to compare with future tests.

Tubing your way to a CT scan

A *CT scan,* also known as a CAT (computerized axial tomography) scan, is a type of x-ray that shows great views of the inside of the cranium. CT scans are used to evaluate for brain disorders (tumors, strokes, head trauma, and acute hemorrhage) or headaches that are the result of chronic sinusitis. The scan is painless. You lie down on a table, and then you are moved into the machine, which is shaped like a gigantic donut. The medical technician performing the procedure is sitting in a separate room, where he watches what's going on via computer monitor and avoids exposure to the radiation. (The dose you are exposed to is considered safe.) During the CT scan, you hear an irritating noise as an x-ray beam takes images each time the machine passes. The images are accumulated and examined by a doctor.

Just because your doctor orders a CT scan, it doesn't mean that you have a brain tumor. When a person does have a brain tumor, an isolated headache as the first and only clinical symptom occurs in only a small percentage (8.2 percent) of patients. (From "Evaluation of Acute Headaches in Adults," by C. Randall Clinch, D.O., *American Family Physician,* February 15, 2001.)

Making magnetic magic with an MRI

MRI (magnetic resonance imaging) can reveal stroke, hemorrhages, skull fractures, malignant diseases, hematomas, sinus problems, tumors, and a number of other problems that may be causing your headaches.

Second-tier tests

Your doctor may ask you to have one or more of the following tests, though using any of these to diagnose headaches is an unlikely scenario.

✔ **Eye pressure test:** This test is used to rule out glaucoma. Doctors can perform this test in one of two ways: by using eye drops to numb your eyes for a short time, or by blowing three puffs of air at the front of each eye. To see the back of your eye more closely, the doctor can put drops in your eyes to *dilate* (make larger) your pupils.

✔ **PET scan (positron emission tomography):** This test uses an imaging technique to view the inside of your head. A PET scan measures brain function and gives the doctor a three-dimensional image to study. When your doctor gives you a PET scan, he asks you to do certain tasks. The PET scan uses low-dose radioactive sugar to measure your brain activity (the amount of radioactivity is roughly equivalent to what you'd get with two chest x-rays). Your doctor then examines the brain areas that show activity when you perform the tasks.

With a PET scan, physicians can also see how a particular drug affects your brain and what happens during your headaches. In fact, the role serotonin plays in the development of a migraine has been supported by PET scans performed during migraineurs' attacks. (The brain chemical serotonin transmits nerve impulses that trigger the release of a substance in the blood vessels that causes pain.)

✔ **Neurological tests:** These tests, which include EEGs (electroencephalograms), focus on detecting epilepsy and other neurological diseases. An EEG isn't effective in identifying types of headaches, but headaches can be indicative of seizures or other abnormalities. Your doctor hopes to rule these abnormalities out with the EEG.

✔ **Sinus CT scan:** Doctors may take sinus CT scans if your headache seems to be caused by sinus problems.

Although CT scanning is more widely available and a little less expensive, MRI is more sensitive in keying in on certain brain abnormalities, such as some brain tumors.

MRI is painless. When you get an MRI, you simply lie down in an enclosed tubelike piece of equipment. (You may have seen an MRI machine on a TV medical drama or documentary).

Most patients have no problem with the close surroundings of the tube. For some, though, a claustrophobic feeling may make them dread this test. If you suffer from *claustrophobia* (a fear of enclosed spaces), your doctor can give you a mild sedative to help you keep calm during the MRI.

If you're totally claustrophobic and dead set against the regular tunnel-type MRI, you can shop around to find a facility that features an *open MRI* (a type of MRI equipment that is not enclosed). The open MRIs are not as widely available as the traditional tunnel-type MRIs, nor are they as accurate.

At some point during your MRI, you may be given an intravenous dye to improve the visual contrast between normal parts of the brain and any abnormalities. If you have ordinary migraines, your MRI will be normal and show no abnormalities.

Even if you have already had an MRI a long time ago, your doctor may still want you to have another one. Your last MRI may have been performed in order to study a different part of your body — or your head or brain may have undergone some changes in the years since.

Limbering up for a lumbar puncture

If your doctor suspects that an *aneurysm* (a ballooning of the wall of a blood vessel) or bleeding from a tangle of blood vessels (AVM) may be the cause of your sudden onset of headaches, he'll probably order a CT scan. If your CT scan is negative (normal), he'll follow it with a lumbar puncture (also known as spinal tap). Negatives on both tests don't completely rule out this serious health condition, because it can take hours for blood to enter the cerebrospinal fluid after hemorrhage occurs.

She likes wide open spaces

A woman who grew up in Texas and was used to wide-open spaces truly didn't want to get into one of those "awful, closed-in things" that they use for MRIs. But she also loathed her debilitating headaches, and her doctor told her the test would help him assess her problem. Still, the thought of getting in the MRI equipment and being "closed in," even for a short period of time, sounded like *Night of the Living Dead* to her.

So she searched around town for an open MRI, but she couldn't find a facility that had one and was also covered by her health insurer. She found herself back at square one.

During a consultation, her headache specialist told her that claustrophobic people usually do just fine if they take a mild sedative prior to their MRI. She decided to give it a try.

On the day of her MRI, she had the first symptoms of a panic attack. The nurse helped her do deep-breathing exercises to calm her anxiety. After the sedative took effect, she was moved into position, and the test was performed without trouble.

She found out that she did have migraines and nothing more serious, so she was glad she had the MRI done.

The purpose of a lumbar puncture is to check for blood in your spinal fluid — cerebrospinal fluid (CSF), to be exact. With a lumbar puncture, your doctor withdraws a sample of the fluid around the brain and spinal cord via a needle that is briefly inserted into your lower back. Patients report discomfort that ranges from mild to painful, but the lumbar puncture is generally well tolerated. A big downside of a lumbar puncture: You may get a headache that can last for hours after the procedure. These headaches occur only when standing, are relieved by lying down, and rarely last for days.

A lumbar puncture can also be used to check for infection or highlight any CSF pressure abnormalities that may be linked to headaches.

Hunkering Down to Come up with a Migraine-Busting Plan

The test results are in, and you're ready for a planning meeting. Now that it's clear that you have migraines, you and your specialist can come up with a migraine-busting plan that will probably feature medications (see Chapters 7 and 8), lifestyle changes (see the chapters in Part IV), and other ideas for quality living (see Chapters 15, 16, and 17).

With a grand-scheme plan, it'll be easier to relegate those pesky migraines to a back burner position in your life, once and for all.

Typically, a migraine plan will include

- ✓ **Dietary fixer-uppers:** You identify and stay away from food triggers that are likely to set off your migraines (see Chapter 11).

- ✓ **Environment upgrade:** You work to reduce your exposure to smell-triggers and environmental toxins (see Chapter 13).

- ✓ **Lifestyle shape-up:** You figure out what types of exercise give rise to your headaches. You also figure out what types of exercise enhance your overall health and help prevent your headaches (see Chapter 12). The latter are the exercises you'll continue to do.

- ✓ **Medications:** With the help of your healthcare provider, you try migraine medications until you zero in on a combative that helps and, if necessary, a preventive that works for you (see Chapters 7 and 8).

- ✓ **Work/home platform:** You discover what to do when the people around you have trouble understanding why you are sometimes disabled by a migraine, and why you sometimes bail on activities (to go home and go to bed — hopefully to sleep your migraine off). See Chapters 16 and 17 for information on coping well with the family and work repercussions of migraines.

Facing insurance stumbling blocks

It's not that your health insurer doesn't want you to get help for your headaches, but you may suspect that someone's plotting against you when you go up against the thorny details of sorting out HMO (health maintenance organization) stumbling blocks. Some common problems you may encounter are

✔ **Getting a referral to a headache specialist:** HMOs may apply pressure on primary care doctors to limit the number of referrals they give. Typically, your primary care doctor will try to diagnose and treat you and hold off on referring you to another doctor, unless you don't show improvement or your symptoms change. However, if your initial symptoms are complicated or worrisome, he may refer you right off the bat.

If your insurance is a PPO (preferred provider organization), you don't need a referral to see a specialist.

If your primary care physician gives you a medication for your symptoms and it doesn't work, and then you go through the same routine a second or third time with different medications, you can ask for a referral to a headache specialist.

✔ **Medication limitations:** Your health insurance company may limit the number of migraine pills it will pay for in a given month. So what happens if you use up your prescription and you're left high and dry?

You can ask your doctor to send a letter of medical necessity to your insurance company. In the letter, he can justify your need for a greater allotment of monthly pain medication. This strategy often works quite well.

✔ **Alternative treatment bans:** Alternative treatments (see Chapter 9) often get a thumbs-down from insurance companies. Using biofeedback and other such options may require you to pay the fees yourself, because it's not likely you'll get your insurer to step up to the plate.

Let your doctor know how you prefer to take your medication. He can prescribe you a pill that dissolves on your tongue, an injection (shot), or a tablet.

You can track your medication intake by keeping a chart of your migraines and their patterns, and the effect of medications on them. (See the headache journal in Chapter 3.)

You know just how good it feels to set yourself up as the Migraine Guru: the one in charge of controlling your headache fate and deciding which treatments you're going to use. At times, it's downright invigorating.

As the Migraine Guru, you can take a proactive stance when dealing with your migraines by

✔ Anticipating how special situations affect you headache-wise

✔ Being a major player in making lifestyle changes that will help prevent migraines (see the chapters in Part IV)

✔ Dealing with work and family in effective ways (see Chapters 16 and 17)

✔ Deciding if you should try a multifaceted approach: a combination of *homeopathic therapy* (stimulating the body to use its powers to heal), traditional medicine, and biofeedback, for example

✔ Weighing in on the alternative options: colonic irrigation, transcutaneous electrical nerve stimulator (TENS), and flickering light therapy. (We don't cover these alternatives, because most of them are unproven. We focus on the remedies that do work.)

If you and your doctor believe that a certain migraine treatment is necessary but your insurance company refuses to approve it, you can appeal the decision in writing to the appeals board of the insurance company. If this strategy fails, you can always hire an attorney. Sometimes a stern letter from a lawyer can get an approval for a treatment that you and your doctor agree is needed. However, don't bother going this route for alternative treatments, because your insurance company probably isn't going to cover them, no matter what you do.

Part III
Giving Migraines a Knockout Punch

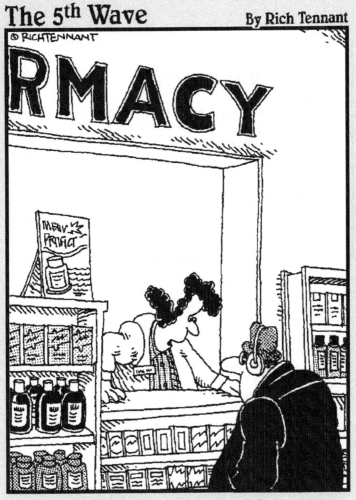

The 5th Wave   By Rich Tennant

"We'll whisper your name when your
migraine medication is ready."

In this part . . .

*P*art III unveils the nitty-gritty on pummeling your pain
via over-the-counter medications and prescription
drugs. Plus, you get the scoop on complementary remedies that some migraine folks use for relieving pain and
warding off headaches — treatments such as biofeedback,
relaxation techniques, acupuncture, and walking. Part III
also features tips on making medical decisions when
you're in a migraine-haze and spotlights emergency-room
tactics.

Chapter 7

Spelling Relief without a Prescription

. . . .

In This Chapter

▶ Trying over-the-counter (OTC) pills

▶ Sidestepping the mistake of overusing OTC drugs

▶ Using vitamin and herbal supplements to fight migraines

. . . .

You have a quandary on your hands: You hate headaches, but you don't like taking prescription drugs. This aversion to drugs is just a personal quirk of yours, but it's a very real concern for you in your search for headache relief.

So, in your crusade to curb migraine pain, you look at non-prescription options, starting with first-tier headache medications — the over-the-counter (OTC) drugs you buy at the drugstore or grocery store. Of course, you can't expect OTC medications to pack the same kind of wallop as a heavy-duty prescription medication, but sometimes a little dab will do you.

You may want to go over the counter at your whole foods/health store and stock up on herbal and vitamin remedies.

In this chapter, we talk about the pros and cons of non-prescription treatments that may be just what the doctor ordered . . . so to speak.

Counting on Over-the-Counter Medications

Some folks just hate prescription drugs. They don't like the way certain drugs made them feel in the past. If you belong to this school of thought, you may be drawn to a less aggressive, over-the-counter (OTC) approach to pain-fighting.

Generally thought of as kinder and gentler than prescription medications, OTC remedies include ibuprofen and acetaminophen, which can usually knock out a relatively mild migraine. Aspirin typically isn't strong enough to provide relief for migraines. (Advil, Excedrin, and Motrin are popular over-the-counter headache relievers.)

Even if you're not adverse to taking prescription drugs, try OTCs first, because they're less apt to sideline you. With OTCs, you're probably not going to get drowsy or woozy to the point where you're unable to work, drive, or cope with your kids. (However, if you have any of the warning signs listed in Chapter 18, forget about using OTCs first, and see a doctor pronto!)

If you're a migraineur who gets relief from OTC medications, good for you. But don't feel discouraged or turn cranky if OTC medications don't do the trick for you. You may need a prescription pain reliever for those times when you experience a truly difficult headache, and that's nothing to be ashamed of.

Comparing benefits

If you have severe migraines, it's pretty unlikely that a medication you can buy over the counter can provide the kind of pain relief you need. But that doesn't mean that you can't try OTC medications — exceptions to every rule do exist. So if you prefer to try OTC medications first, you definitely should.

People may tell you otherwise, but it's actually possible for some migraine sufferers to overcome their pain without prescription medication. According to the National Headache Foundation Web site (www.headaches.org), about 60 percent of migraine sufferers use OTC remedies exclusively to manage their headaches.

Sometimes OTC remedies fail to provide you with any type of relief. Other times, they may provide you with a little relief — enough to help you handle the discomfort until your headache is completely resolved with sleep or another dose of the medicine later in the day. If you're one of the lucky ones, you may even find an OTC drug that works very well almost every time you get a headache.

But if your headache is "killing" you, and OTC pills aren't helping, OTC remedies will seem about as effective as tying a banana peel to your forehead (a custom, in some cultures, that produces a cool look but is worthless as pain-relief).

By the way, if you take an OTC tablet referred to as a "migraine formula," don't think that you're practically taking a prescription drug. The truth is that migraine formulas are no stronger than their sibling over-the-counter medications. The FDA (U.S. Food and Drug Administration) allows drug companies to label their products as migraine formulas even though they often don't provide any extra benefits for migraine sufferers.

Get me to the pills on time!

Camilla Pierce, a Houston homemaker and a migraine sufferer for 30 years, explains what works for her: "I've never really known for sure what triggers my headaches exactly, except for any intense physical activity like aerobics — and that always does. I do know that any headache I had would get very bad if left untreated. The only thing that has ever worked for me is Excedrin. I've never had to use any kind of prescription medications for my migraines."

Take OTC pain meds early in your migraine attack, but don't take them often. Don't exceed recommended dosages!

If you take OTC pills for more than two days each week, you may make your pain situation worse. Unfortunately, you may have to wait two or three hours for an OTC drug to relieve your pain. This delay may tempt you to pop more pills in hopes of a quicker resolution. But you must avoid the trap of taking OTC drugs too often; if you're not careful, you may experience increased side effects (stomach upset) or get a rebound headache, which can evolve into a very painful problem (see Chapter 4).

Don't take a caffeine-containing OTC drug on a daily basis, or you may wind up with a caffeine-withdrawal headache when you try to cut back on the pills. If you're having daily headaches, you need to see a doctor for an evaluation and help in setting up a migraine-fighting plan.

If OTCs don't help relieve your migraines, you may need to move up to the next rung on the pain-killing ladder — prescription migraine meds (see Chapter 8). Or you can try supplementing your OTC medications with alternative remedies (see Chapter 9).

Finding anti-inflammatories helpful

Nonsteroidal anti-inflammatory drugs (NSAIDs) are widely used for painful ailments. They come in both prescription and OTC form. The OTC forms include Advil and Motrin (ibuprofen), Aleve (naproxen sodium), and Bayer (aspirin). All of these OTC drugs can have side effects, including stomach irritation and bleeding, nausea, and vomiting.

Excedrin Migraine and Excedrin Extra Strength are staples for many people who have mild-to-moderate migraines (both contain exactly the same meds). The common side effect — stomach upset — may be an acceptable tradeoff for pain relief.

If you're taking Extra-Strength Excedrin or Excedrin Migraine, you're using a product that combines acetaminophen and aspirin with caffeine. With Aspirin-Free Excedrin, you're taking acetaminophen and caffeine — a combination that can provide pain relief for some migraineurs.

Assuming that you're an adult who's not allergic to NSAIDs (see Chapter 8 for more info on NSAIDs) or any of the ingredients in Excedrin, and that you're not pregnant, you may use it as your staple ammo for most headaches. Then, on the rare occasion when the going gets rough — and a headache turns into Bad Bad Leroy Brown — you may need to turn to your tougher backup: a prescription migraine troubleshooter.

Admiring Advil

When taken early in a migraine attack, Advil may work well in relieving the pain of a mild migraine.

To stop an in-progress migraine, you can try Advil Migraine. Mild to moderate migraines often respond well to Advil Migraine, which is exactly the same as Advil Liqui-Gels. Both work faster than garden-variety Advil.

Sidestepping the Side Effects of Too Many OTC Drugs

Take too many OTC drugs, and you may be doomed to experience side effects such as nausea, vomiting, or the Eternal Headache, better known as a rebound headache (see Chapter 4). Furthermore, excessive OTC drug use can result in problems such as liver or kidney damage (depending on the medication).

So aim to be a savvy migraineur and safeguard yourself from overdosing. If you're using OTC remedies for a very bad migraine, find a way to keep track of the number of pills you're taking. If you're reaching for the pill bottle in the middle of the night — when you're half-asleep and reeling from pain — you may get confused and take more than you should (unless you have some kind of system for keeping track).

One woman tells of setting out her just-in-case migraine pills at the start of her headaches so that she won't surpass the number that's safe to take in a 24-hour period. She uses a chart to help her remember when she took the first one, when it's okay to take another, and so on.

This advice may sound like simple connect-the-dots guidance, but the truth is, you can use all the help you can get when a pain stupor mutes your thinking processes. (You know this if you've been there.) And if a mate or friend isn't standing by to hand out pills, you better find your own way to deal with pain relievers in a safe manner.

As a general rule, you may be inviting disaster (a rebound headache; see Chapter 4) if you're taking the recommended dosage of a medication two to three days a week for several weeks.

Using Vitamin and Herbal Supplements

Vitamin supplements work well for many people who battle migraines. Because some headache experts now believe that a lack of sufficient magnesium is the culprit behind many migraines, the practice of smart-bombing migraines with supplements has become popular. Other vitamins can be used to bring balance to your body so that it's better able to combat migraines.

By the same token, some people are big fans of treating migraines with herbal remedies — a controversial option on which the jury is still out. You're probably not going to find many physicians who'll give herbal remedies a hearty thumbs-up. Not yet, anyway, because studies to illustrate that these supplements are safe and effective have been insufficient.

If you're going to use vitamins and herbal supplements to help treat your migraines, you should be supervised by a doctor, and perhaps even a nutritionist. You need to have a healthcare provider look at your entire health picture before you start taking a few fish-oil capsules here, a little magnesium there, and a few leaves of feverfew for a snack. Remember that every part of your headache game plan needs to mesh neatly for the best overall pain-fighting effect. Remedies that aren't compatible can add some new symptoms to your troubles.

Some migraine researchers believe that certain vitamin supplements can decrease your likelihood of developing headaches by balancing your system. Therefore, some migraineurs who are thrashing around for pain relief get very excited about the idea of taking vitamin supplements as a migraine remedy.

Taking your vitamins

While vitamin advocates — and many doctors — support using vitamins to help get rid of migraines, many healthcare providers aren't convinced that nutritional supplements are beneficial for treating migraines. Also, the excessive use of vitamins sometimes can result in nasty side effects: Too much vitamin B6 can cause numbness in your hands and mouth; an overdose of magnesium supplements may affect your nervous system adversely, and magnesium intoxication can be fatal; and too much vitamin C can give you diarrhea.

Avoiding ephedrine

A headache is but one of many problems/symptoms that can result from taking supplements containing ephedrine. The U.S. Department of Health and Human Services warns consumers not to take dietary supplements containing ephedrine, because these products pose significant health risks, but they continue to be popular among health-club enthusiasts.

Marketed as weight-loss products and alternatives to illegal street drugs such as ecstasy, these supplements contain botanical (or so-called *natural*) sources of *ephedrine* — an amphetamine-like stimulant that can have dangerous effects on the heart and nervous system.

These products are marketed under many brand names, and labels promise or suggest that they can promote weight loss, produce euphoria, enhance sexual sensations, heighten energy, and so on. But these supplements may cause possible adverse effects that range from headache, dizziness, and heart palpitations to heart attack, stroke, seizures, psychosis, and death.

So stay away from products that contain ephedrine, which may be listed under one of many aliases: ma huang, Chinese ephedra, ma huang extract, ephedra, ephedra sinica, ephedra extract, ephedra herb powder, or epitonin.

If you suspect that you have overdosed on vitamins, go to an emergency room or call your doctor. Some signs of vitamin overdose include:

- Cloudy urine
- Convulsions
- Dry lips and skin
- Frequent urination
- Irritability
- Itchy skin
- Lack of appetite
- Mood swings
- Muscle weakness

It's a good idea to seek help when attempting to vitamin-bomb your migraines. Headache specialists are good sources for advice on vitamin supplementation. They're up-to-date on the latest studies, and they have experience monitoring patients who use supplements for migraine treatment.

Correcting dietary deficiencies may help your migraines as well as your overall health. Before you try any of the following supplements, get a doctor's advice on what supplements may be best for you (and what supplements will work with the medications you're already taking). Your physician takes into consideration your age, past medical history, your current food regimen, and other factors that should go into the mix when deciding what supplements you need for deficiencies. But try to get most of your vitamins and minerals from food. Too many vitamins can be as dangerous as a deficiency of vitamins.

With each of the following supplements, the dose listed is the recommended daily dose for adults *(mg is an abbreviation for milligrams)*. You can try using these supplements for your headaches, but if you experience negative side effects, back off on supplementation. You don't want to take vitamins that make you feel worse instead of better. (Incidentally, vitamin E is measured in IUs, or international units.)

- **Magnesium (400 mg):** Magnesium can be depleted by medications such as diuretics (called water pills because they reduce the amount of water in the body), alcohol consumption, and chronic medical problems such as diabetes. But if you eat spinach, nuts, bananas, bran, and whole-grain breads and cereals, you may get plenty of magnesium without taking a supplement. Symptoms of taking too much magnesium include diarrhea, drowsiness, and lethargy.

- **B2 (400 mg):** Studies have shown that 400 mg of vitamin B2 (riboflavin) can greatly reduce migraine frequency. One rare bothersome side effect of vitamin B2 is diarrhea.

- **Fish-oil concentrate pills (2,000 mg):** Fish-oil pills with 360 mg of the omega-3 fatty acid EPA (eicosapentaenoic acid) and 240 mg of the omega-3 fatty acid DHA (docosahexaenoic acid) are believed to reduce the intensity of an existing headache or help stave off headaches so that you don't have them as often.

- **Vitamin C (2,000 mg):** These supplements are usually sold in 1,000 and 1,500 mg pills, so you can take two of the 1,000 mg pills a day. Vitamin C is recommended for headache prevention.

- **Vitamin E (400 IU):** Vitamin E is good for circulation, and thus, helpful for some people who suffer from migraines.

- **Vitamin B6 (200 mg):** Some researchers think that vitamin B6 helps to ward off headaches. (Don't exceed the recommended dose.)

Tiptoeing through the herbal remedies

Herbal remedies are occasionally used as adjuncts to a central migraine-management plan. On the other hand, some people claim that certain herbs take care of their migraine pain entirely! (If someone swears by an herbal-only approach, check for a crystal ball and gypsy jewelry, because getting rid of a full-fledged migraine with nothing but herbal remedies ranks right up there with cleaning up an oil spill with tissues.)

If you're working on a migraine management plan, and you're considering some form of herbal supplementation, be sure to consult with your healthcare provider.

Don't imbibe gallons of the hottest gimmick coming down the pike until studies have proven its effectiveness. Remember, one person's anecdotal experience isn't enough to gamble your head on. Maybe the latest buzz around the water cooler is that drinking powdered ginger and water cures migraines! Hip-hip-hooray! But, on the other hand, some miracle migraine myth is spread among the populace just about every other day. Sure, the ginger cure may turn out to be true. Then again, it may be bogus.

Kava (or *kava-kava*) was all hot-cha-cha until there were reports that this herbal remedy made from the plant Piper methysticum may cause liver damage. However, you may still find kava for sale, and it may be labeled as a migraine remedy.

Herbal products aren't regulated for purity, so there can be variability in the amount of herb and impurities present.

If you just can't resist trendy remedies, check with your healthcare provider before taking them. If she gives you the go-ahead, you may want to sample some of the following herbal hotties:

- **Bayberry tea:** Some people use a cup of this drink as a headache deterrent when they feel a migraine coming on. If you still develop a headache after drinking it, try drinking another cup later in the day.

- **Chamomile tea:** This tea is a popular herbal treatment used to relieve migraine pain after a headache hits. It does double duty, as it also helps sooth rocky stomach woes. Drink one or two cups.

- **Feverfew:** Long used as dry leaves in tea to treat inflammation and swelling, and highly lauded as a migraine preventive, feverfew (the herb Tanacetum parthenium) reportedly helps many people. It's usually taken in capsule form. Follow the recommendations on the bottle for dosage.

  Feverfew doesn't work for everyone (of course, neither does anything else). When you stop taking it, you may get jittery and have trouble sleeping for a while.

- **Ginkgo:** Ginkgo biloba, believed to improve blood flow to the brain, may help relieve your headaches.

  Don't use ginkgo if you take anticoagulants (blood thinners), aspirin, lithium, or ergotamine with caffeine. Check with your doctor before using this or any other herbal remedy.

- **Lam Kam Sang Heklin:** This big ol' raw-herb hodgepodge is said to relieve migraines fast.

✔ **St. John's wort:** The herb St. John's wort (Hypericum perforatum) is sometimes used to reduce anxiety and depression and relieve headaches.

Don't use St. John's wort if you're on birth control pills or prescription antidepressants, such as Paxil or Zoloft.

✔ **Valerian:** This herb is used for both anxiety relief and migraine pain relief. Keep doses low, because too much can make you hyperactive.

Using herbal remedies for migraine relief is very controversial. Most people think that for every person who gets help via an herbal remedy, there's another who tried the same thing and got no help whatsoever. (Could it just be a placebo effect?) The same thing can be said of acetaminophen or ibuprofen, although many studies have proven these medications to be effective. One person's surefire solution may be another person's live toad on the head.

Chapter 8

Taking Care of Pain with Prescription Drugs

. . . .

. . . .

*T*oday, doctors have a huge arsenal of headache drugs that can prevent a migraine from getting worse, stop head pain in its tracks, make recurrences less likely, and even prevent a migraine from happening in the first place.

Because a migraineur's brain has overly sensitive circuits that overreact to stimuli that don't bother non-migraine folks, calming down these mega-sensitive nerve cells clearly is critical to pain relief. And that became the job description of a migraine-combating drug that gained U.S. approval in 1993 — sumatriptan. Its success unleashed the drug class of triptans, which have provided tremendous relief for many migraineurs in the decade since.

But finding relief isn't always simple. Because migraines are very individualistic in pain level and frequency, and because people respond differently to different medications, you may have to try several prescription medicines to find the one that works well for you. You must hang in there until you find the right stuff, because the migraine-pain-relief options today are amazingly effective, and you have everything to gain from taking the time to zero in on your solution.

In this chapter, you find everything you ever wanted to know about various drugs for migraines. We familiarize you with their impact on headaches, their side effects, their likelihood to cause dependency, and their incompatibility with other meds and health conditions.

Looking for Relief in All the Right Places

Sometimes you get tired of hearing yourself repeat the same old refrain: "My head's killing me!" But it's hard to come up with creative phrases when you're writhing in pain (and perhaps nauseated, as well). The truth is, a migraine makes you desperate for answers, and your battle cry becomes the oft-repeated "Help me get rid of this head-splitting agony!"

So you turn to your doctor, and he introduces a whole field of dreamy medications designed to eliminate migraine pain. The only problem is, what works for one person may not necessarily work for you. So trial and error is the name of the migraine-med-sorting game.

The process starts when you huddle with your migraine-specialist doctor (see Chapters 5 and 6), and the two of you firm up a determination to devise a headache management plan — with both drug and nondrug remedies — that will help you ward off headaches before they take up residence in your skull, or fight them after they move in.

Remember that no book can be a substitute for an in-person, one-on-one consultation with your personal physician, who knows all about your particular medical needs and conditions. Don't skip the consultation process!

Just to keep things interesting, the guide that many doctors use as a reference on drugs — a monthly booklet called *Monthly Prescribing Reference* — has a comment at the start of its migraine-drug coverage that says, essentially, that no one really knows for sure exactly how migraines work, so the way that many anti-migraine drugs work is only theoretical, and this is especially true when it comes to combination products.

The name game

Understand that each drug has several names associated with it — not just to confuse you but to flesh out the persona and character of the particular drug. For example, a given medication has a chemical name that's rarely used but is reflective of its chemical composition, a descriptive class name, a generic (hard-to-pronounce) name that points to the drug family it came from, and a *trade name* — the registered name the manufacturer gives the drug — which is probably the one you're most familiar with. Some examples of trade names are Imitrex and Advil.

In the same way that you can call an automobile by a descriptive name (a steel, plastic, rubber, and chrome, human-steered, gasoline-powered vehicle), generic name (car), or trade name (BMW), you can also sort a medicine by its descriptive class name (serotonin receptor agonist), generic name (rizatriptan), and finally, its trade name (Maxalt). The true chemical name for a drug, which is usually a mile long, doesn't come up very often — fortunately.

The information on migraine medications provided in this chapter is intended primarily for people who don't have special medical conditions in addition to their migraines, those who aren't 65 or older, and those who aren't children. If you fall into one of these groups, consult your physician for advice on appropriate ways to treat your migraines. (See Chapter 20 on children, and Chapter 23 on seniors.)

Always check with a doctor before taking any drug! Don't take other people's headache remedies or improvise on your own medications. You must beware of any unusual migraine, because it may signal a more dangerous condition, such as brain hemorrhage, aneurysm, meningitis, or another life-threatening condition.

Generalizing about drug types

In your investigation of drug therapies, you'll find that the arsenal of anti-migraine drugs features quite a variety, including the following:

- General pain-fighters
- Drugs that address migraine side effects
- Medicines made especially for migraines
- Medications that were originally created for other medical conditions but were found to help migraine pain, as well

The two overall categories for migraine-treating drugs are *abortives*, medicines that stop a headache that's already under way, and *prophylactics* (or *preventives*), drugs aimed at preventing a migraine from occurring. Prophylactics, by the way, aren't the first line of defense, simply because you don't want to take medication that you don't need — and a regimen of preventives requires a daily tablet in most cases.

Coming to terms with migraines

Certain words keep popping up in headache talks — so much so, that you really need to know migraine jargon to stay abreast of what's going on in the ever-changing treatment field.

To sort through all the pain relievers, though, you need to understand their "doctor names" — because physicians tend to toss these names about during headache-treatment talks. Take a look at the following list of common pain relievers:

- ✔ **Abortives (or abortive therapy):** Medications called abortives fight existing migraines. These pain relievers are also called acute medication, rescue meds, and relief drugs. They work to relieve pain after a headache arrives, whether it's just warming up or blasting your head like a rock concert. This category includes plenty of prescription drugs, as well as some first-line-of-defense OTCs (over-the-counter medications) such as Excedrin Migraine and Advil Migraine (see Chapter 7 for OTCs).

- ✔ **Antidepressants:** Certain antidepressants, which are frequently used to treat depression, have found a second role as migraine preventives. Some of these are Elavil and Pamelor.

- ✔ **Antiemetics:** These medications are used to control migraine-associated nausea and vomiting, but they can also help relieve migraine pain itself. Two antiemetics are Reglan and Phenergan (see "Getting Nausea Relief," later in this chapter).

- ✔ **Beta blockers:** These drugs, long used to treat high blood pressure, can also be used to prevent migraines. Examples are Inderal and Blocadren.

- ✔ **Calcium channel blockers:** Commonly used to treat people with high blood pressure, calcium channel blockers also work for preventing migraines, because they can establish a balance in your blood vessels and stave off oxygen deficit in the brain. Calan is an example.

- ✔ **Ergotamine:** The drugs called ergotamines, or ergot derivatives, can abort acute migraines because they constrict blood vessels, but more importantly, they block pain impulses from getting to the brain. In other words, this kind of drug causes a narrowing of the brain's arteries and diminishes pain. Examples of ergotamine-based medications are Cafergot, Ergostat, Migranal, DHE-45, and Sansert.

- ✔ **Monoamine oxidase inhibitors (MAOIs):** The MAOIs are antidepressants that are used for migraine prevention. Doctors don't usually choose MAOIs as the first line of defense, because they have the potential for interacting with so many different medications and foods, which can result in serious health consequences. If your headaches don't respond to other prophylactic treatments, your doctor may prescribe an MAOI. Examples of MAOIs are Nardil, Parnate, and Marplan.

- ✔ **Narcotic analgesics:** These medications contain an opioid (a drug that acts on the body just like opium and its derivatives), and therefore, they aren't available over the counter, but they can be used for severe headache pain. (These are different from regular analgesics described in Chapter 7.) Some opium-like compounds that are sometimes used for pain relief are butorphanol and oxycodone.

- ✔ **Nonsteroidal anti-inflammatory drugs (NSAIDs):** These are painkillers that people take for a number of medical conditions, including mild to moderate headaches. Used to address (and reduce) the inflammation that occurs during a headache, NSAIDs inhibit the production of *prostaglandins,* hormone-like substances that are known to cause pain. Some of the NSAIDs are Aleve, ibuprofen, and aspirin.

If you're pregnant or breastfeeding, ask your doctor before using NSAIDs. NSAIDs should not be used during the third trimester of pregnancy, because there's the possibility that the use of such drugs can affect the baby's heart. However, you can take acetaminophen during pregnancy.

- **Preventives or prophylactics:** You really have to love these meds, because they're the ones that can decrease the frequency of your headaches and perhaps even prevent them from showing up at all. Hooray! On the other hand, they don't work if an attack is already underway.

  Preventives include prescription drugs and OTC drugs such as naproxen. You shouldn't start yourself on a daily regimen of preventive medication — treatment with preventives should be initiated by your doctor. Prophylactics include: beta blockers, antidepressants, anticonvulsants, and calcium antagonists.

- **Selective serotonin reuptake inhibitors (SSRIs):** The SSRIs are common antidepressants and antianxiety medications that can interact badly with some migraine medications, such as the triptans, and cause complications. Examples of SSRIs are Prozac (also available as the generic fluoxetine), Paxil, Zoloft, Celexa, Luvox, and Lexapro.

- **Triptans:** This term refers to medications that end with "triptan," such as the medicine sumatriptan. These prescription meds are often used as initial treatment for migraines.

Some of the nondrug terms your doctor may throw around include:

- **5-HT:** This is serotonin, a chemical released in the brain that transmits signals between nerve cells and can affect the blood vessels in your head. Researchers believe that this substance plays a prominent role in migraine attacks because a narrowing of vessels (via serotonin) curbs head pain by blocking pain impulses from getting to the brain.

- **Caffeine:** Though harmful when overused (and the actual villain in caffeine withdrawal headaches), caffeine is only a trigger when someone gets too much, and then it can cause a headache. Otherwise, it constricts blood vessels and thus relieves pain.

- **Serotonin:** The fluctuations of this brain chemical are involved in migraine development.

- **Vasodilation:** When blood vessels increase in size.

- **Vasoconstriction:** When blood vessels decrease in size.

Finding Out What to Expect and How You React

When you get a prescription, ask your doctor to explain fully what to expect when you take the medication he prescribed. Pain relief? Nausea relief? Does the drug have side effects, such as sleepiness or anxiety? (See information on side effects in the "Fighting Back: Abortive Medications for Migraines Underway" and "Stopping Migraines Upfront: Prophylactics" sections, later in this chapter.)

When you take the prescribed medication, monitor your reactions to it. People react differently to different drugs. You're the best judge of how well your body is responding to a particular drug. Be sure to check with your doctor if you have any questions, or if you have concerns about certain symptoms.

Of course, you have to be realistic. You want pain relief from the remedy, so you may have to put up with a side effect or two — but you don't want a set of brand-new symptoms that are worse than the headache! Examples of bad signs are: mental effects such as depression or mood swings, or debilitating physical drawbacks such as diarrhea.

The point is, you want to be a savvy consumer when assessing your migraine medication. The Migraine Pain-Relief Mall features scads of options, so you don't have to settle for one that doesn't work well or makes you feel "sick."

Fighting Back: Abortive Medications for Migraines Underway

You have a headache, you're hurting, and you want it to go away. This is where abortive drugs come in — they're the medications that can give an existing migraine a knockout punch. These pain relievers aren't intended for headache prevention.

Many abortive drugs can't be used for hemiplegic or basilar migraines. Hemiplegic migraines can cause temporary paralysis on one side of the body. If you have basilar migraines, you usually feel pain on the back of your head, and you may experience frightening symptoms, such as slurred speech, confusion, lack of coordination, nausea, double vision, vertigo, and even a loss of consciousness. This kind of headache can cause stroke, coma, and, sometimes, death. If you suspect that you have either of these headaches types, you should have your doctor evaluate you to rule out the possibility that your symptoms are indications of something worse. (See Chapter 4 for more on these headache types.)

The format used in the drug section is the brand name first, with the generic drug name in parentheses. In each category, we describe a sample drug (or drugs) in detail — one(s) commonly prescribed.

Follow your doctor's instructions on dosing. Don't take more (or less) medication than you're supposed to.

Nonsteroidal anti-inflammatory drugs (NSAIDs)

Often used for chronic pain, the NSAIDs are popular migraine remedies that come in both over-the-counter and prescription versions. These medications are actually used for both abortive and prophylactic treatment of migraines. Possible side effects include diarrhea, nausea, and stomach bleeding. Some examples are Advil, Motrin, Naprosyn, and aspirin.

Naprosyn (naproxen)

Naprosyn is often used to relieve the pain of menstrual cramps and arthritis, as well as mild to moderate migraines. Aleve, Naprelan, and Anaprox also contain the same generic medication naproxen, but their dosing is different.

- ✔ **Mode of delivery:** Tablet.

- ✔ **Possible side effects:** Abdominal pain, peptic ulcers, gastrointestinal bleeding, heartburn, nausea, and sleepiness. Taking more than the recommended amount of Naprosyn can cause problems such as vomiting, drowsiness, and heartburn.

- ✔ **Don't use if:** You have had a bad reaction to aspirin, Naprosyn, or any other NSAID in the past. Don't take Naprosyn if you're pregnant or breastfeeding, you have liver or kidney disease, you have a history of ulcers, you take blood thinners, or you have clotting problems.

- ✔ **Doesn't react well with:** Aspirin, other NSAIDs, or blood thinners. Naprosyn also interacts with other medications, so be sure to check with your doctor.

Triptans

A group of drugs that totally transformed the treatment of migraines because of their amazing effectiveness, the triptans appear to affect a certain serotonin receptor in your brain that results in the constriction of blood vessels, but more importantly, they block pain impulses from getting to the brain. Possible side effects include dizziness, chest pain, and anxiety. Some examples are Amerge, Zomig, and Imitrex.

You shouldn't take triptans if you have cardiovascular disease (heart disease). And, unless your doctor evaluates you and suggests otherwise, you shouldn't take triptans if you have major risk factors for heart disease (such as diabetes, obesity, high cholesterol, high blood pressure, or a family history of heart disease), you smoke, you're pregnant or breastfeeding, you're postmenopausal, you're a man over 40 years old, or you're a woman older than 65.

In one study of 43 hospital employees, researchers at the Georgia Headache Treatment Center in Augusta, Georgia, compared patients using their regular therapy for 12 to 18 weeks followed by injections of sumatriptan as needed for migraine pain for six months. The number of migraine days patients got pain relief by using sumatriptan was 75 percent, whereas it was only 25 percent with their usual therapy. Lost workplace productivity (and non-workplace activity time) was 35 percent lower with sumatriptan therapy. This figure underscores the finding that treating migraines with sumatriptan improves pain relief, reduces lost workplace productivity and non-workplace activity time, and enhances quality of life.

The triptans can be used to relieve migraine headaches with or without aura, but they shouldn't be used for unusual types of migraine, such as basilar or hemiplegic migraine.

Amerge (naratriptan)

Amerge works for a longer period of time than the other triptans, so it works well if you have trouble with recurrence of headaches. This medication is commonly used for migraines with or without aura, and it's often prescribed for menstrual migraines. You may take it any time after your symptoms begin.

- ✔ **Mode of delivery:** Tablet.

- ✔ **Possible side effects:** Nausea, dizziness, drowsiness, and fatigue. Although rare, serious cardiac problems may also result.

- ✔ **Don't use if:** You have basilar or hemiplegic migraine (see headache types in Chapter 4), heart disease, uncontrolled high blood pressure, a history of *TIA* (a transient ischemic attack is an episode of neurological dysfunction resembling a stroke, but that resolves completely) or stroke, liver or kidney problems, or if you've taken other triptans or ergotamine-type drugs within the previous 24 hours.

- ✔ **Doesn't react well with:** SSRIs, ergotamine-type medicines, or triptans. Also, don't use in addition to other triptans you've taken within 24 hours.

Frova (frovatriptan succinate)

Frova, which became available in early 2002, is the newest triptan to receive FDA approval for the treatment of migraines in adults.

✔ **Mode of delivery:** Tablet.

✔ **Possible side effects:** Fatigue, flushing, dizziness, dry mouth, chest and throat tightness, and, rarely, serious cardiac problems.

✔ **Don't use if:** You have heart disease, a history of stroke or TIA, uncontrolled high blood pressure, or you have taken other triptans or ergotamine-type drugs within the previous 24 hours. Don't use for basilar or hemiplegic migraine.

If you have liver problems or risk factors for heart disease, or if you're elderly, pregnant, or breastfeeding, your doctor will consider whether there's a better medication for you.

✔ **Doesn't react well with:** Other triptans, SSRIs, methysergide, or ergotamines.

Imitrex (sumatriptan)

Known as an excellent first-line therapy, Imitrex even works on tough headaches that are hard to shake. It can be used for acute migraines but not for basilar or hemiplegic migraines. You should take Imitrex when symptoms first appear, but it may also be used any time during an attack. You often get relief within an hour or two.

✔ **Modes of delivery:** Tablet, nasal spray, injection.

✔ **Possible side effects:** Flushing, muscle weakness, dizziness, sore throat, drowsiness, neck pain, anxiety, agitation, headaches, itching, chest pain, sweating, and, rarely, seizures and serious cardiac problems.

Too much Imitrex may cause such problems as sluggishness, tremors, or seizures.

✔ **Don't use if:** You have a history of heart disease, heart attack, angina, strokes, or TIAs, you have basilar or hemiplegic migraine, uncontrolled high blood pressure, or liver problems, or you've taken ergot-type drugs or any other triptans within the previous 24 hours or MAOIs within the last two weeks.

If you're at high risk for heart disease (such as being obese or having diabetes, high blood pressure, or a family history of heart disease), you have kidney problems, or you're pregnant or breastfeeding, your doctor will consider whether there's a better medicine for you.

✔ **Doesn't interact well with:** MAOIs (such as Nardil), ergotamine-containing drugs (such as Cafergot), or the SSRI antidepressants (such as Prozac and Zoloft). Don't use Imitrex if you've taken any other triptan within 24 hours.

Maxalt (rizatriptan)

Maxalt is laudable for working soon after you take it, often within an hour or two. The orally disintegrating tablet form can be taken without water, because it melts on your tongue. Rizatriptan comes in both Maxalt-MLT (the melting tablet form) and Maxalt.

- ✔ **Mode of delivery:** Tablet (common tablet form and orally disintegrating tablet form).

- ✔ **Possible side effects:** Sleepiness, chest pressure, dizziness, nausea, fatigue, and, rarely, serious cardiac problems.

- ✔ **Don't use if:** You have heart disease, uncontrolled high blood pressure, basilar or hemiplegic migraine, or you've taken ergotamine-type drugs or other triptans within the previous 24 hours or MAOIs within the previous two weeks.

  If you are pregnant or breastfeeding, have risk factors for heart disease (such as diabetes, obesity, or smoking), or have liver or kidney problems, your doctor will consider whether there's a better medication for you.

- ✔ **Doesn't interact well with:** SSRIs, MAOIs, methysergide, ergotamines, or other triptans. When taking propranolol, your dose of Maxalt should be lowered (consult your doctor).

Zomig (zolmitriptan)

Zomig is a triptan that works fast and, for some people, helps relieve nausea.

- ✔ **Mode of delivery:** Tablet (common tablet form and orally disintegrating tablet form).

- ✔ **Possible side effects:** Dizziness, nausea, skin tingling, dry mouth, cold or warm sensation, drowsiness, weakness, trouble swallowing, chest or throat tightness, and, rarely, serious cardiac problems. Too much Zomig may make you feel sleepy.

- ✔ **Don't use if:** You have a history of heart disease, angina, or heart attack, uncontrolled high blood pressure, or you have taken ergot-type drugs or other triptans within the previous 24 hours or MAOIs within the previous two weeks. You should also avoid using Zomig if you have risk factors for heart disease (such as smoking, diabetes, or you're overweight), an irregular heartbeat, liver problems, or you're pregnant or breastfeeding. Don't take this medication for basilar or hemiplegic migraine.

- ✔ **Doesn't interact well with:** MAOIs, SSRIs, ergotamine-type drugs, or other triptans. Some drugs (Tylenol, birth control pills, Tagamet, and others) interact with Zomig, so check with your doctor before taking it.

Other triptans include Axert (almotriptan) and Relpax (eletriptan).

Always check with your doctor for interactions with any medications you're taking.

Combination drugs

Named because they are, indeed, combinations of several drugs, combination medications often work well on migraines. Some examples of combination drugs are Fiorinal, Esgic, and Midrin.

All combination drugs have the potential to make you feel sleepy. You shouldn't drink alcohol when taking these pills. And you must be careful not to exceed the recommended dosage (exceeding the dosage can lead to rebound headaches, see Chapter 4). The side effects of combo drugs may include the worsening of your headaches (if you use combination drugs too often) and possibly drug dependency.

Midrin (isometheptene mucate, dichloralphenazone, acetaminophen)

Midrin, which contains isometheptene, acetaminophen, and dichloralphenazone, serves to narrow dilated blood vessels that have been implicated in migraine pain. Midrin is commonly used for the treatment of mild-to-moderate migraines and menstrual migraines. You take it when you first notice symptoms.

- ✔ **Mode of delivery:** Capsule.
- ✔ **Possible side effects:** Dizziness, sleepiness, and rash.
- ✔ **Don't use if:** You have hypersensitivity to any of the components of Midrin (check the ingredients in the medication's literature), glaucoma, uncontrolled high blood pressure, severe kidney disease, liver disease, or heart disease, you've taken MAOIs within the previous two weeks, or you have had a stroke or heart attack. If you have high blood pressure, peripheral vascular disease, or are pregnant or breastfeeding, your doctor may want to consider other medication options.
- ✔ **Doesn't interact well with:** MAOIs and blood thinners. Also, be aware that Midrin's sedative effect can be increased if you take antihistamines, Valium, or another central nervous system depressant. Avoid taking Midrin with alcohol.

Ergotamine derivatives

Made from a fungus, these drugs constrict blood vessels in your brain. They sometimes cause vomiting, nausea, and muscle cramps. Some examples of ergotamine derivatives are Migranal, Cafergot, and DHE-45.

Cafergot (contains ergotamine tartrate and caffeine)

Cafergot can be used for migraines with or without aura. Take it when symptoms of a migraine first appear.

- ✔ **Modes of delivery:** Suppository, tablet.

- ✔ **Possible side effects:** Severe vomiting, elevated blood pressure, nausea, slow or fast heartbeat, numbness, weakness, chest pain, and muscle pain. Too much Cafergot may cause convulsions, headaches, leg pain, coldness in your extremities, high or low blood pressure, vomiting, coma, or drug dependency. Ergot poisoning can be a very serious matter.

- ✔ **Don't use if:** You have kidney or liver disease, high blood pressure, heart disease, peripheral vascular disease, allergy to drugs that contain caffeine or ergotamine, or you're pregnant or breastfeeding.

- ✔ **Doesn't interact well with:** Sudafed or any drug that causes blood vessels to constrict, nicotine or nicotine drugs that are used for smoking cessation, beta-blocker drugs (such as propranolol), or certain antibiotics (consult your doctor).

Migranal (dihydroergotamine mesylate)

This ergotamine-containing nasal spray provides pain relief by altering the amount of serotonin in your brain and constricting blood vessels. It contains the same active ingredient as the injectable form DHE-45. Migranal is a good drug choice for combating migraines that keep coming back. Don't use Migranal for hemiplegic or basilar migraines.

- ✔ **Mode of delivery:** Nasal spray.

- ✔ **Possible side effects:** Dizziness, drowsiness, nausea, vomiting, nasal congestion, heart problems, and hot flushes. Too much Migranal may cause ergot-poisoning symptoms such as headaches, convulsions, muscle pain, numbness, or cold extremities.

- ✔ **Don't take if:** You have basilar or hemiplegic migraine, heart disease (including angina), uncontrolled high blood pressure, liver or kidney disease, blood vessel problems (such as Raynaud's phenomenon), you've taken triptans or other ergot-type medications within the previous 24 hours or MAOIs within the previous two weeks, or if you're pregnant or breastfeeding.

- ✔ **Doesn't interact well with:** Other ergotamines, vasoconstrictors, triptans, MAOIs, and erythromycin. Migranal can also interact with multiple other medications, so let your doctor know all of the medicines you're taking. You should also let your doctor know if you have hypothyroidism, because Migranal may adversely affect this condition.

DHE-45 has the same active ingredient as Migranal. It's used for aborting severe headaches in a hurry. It's often given in injection form in emergency rooms to treat long-lasting migraines.

Corticosteroids

Usually the court of last resort for headaches that just won't go away, the corticosteroids mute your body's inflammation response. Possible side effects include anxiety and insomnia. Prednisone is one example of a corticosteroid (see "Calling on Superhero Medications," later in this chapter).

Opioids (or narcotics)

These powerhouse painkillers are usually reserved for terrible migraine pain that won't go away after trying less potent pills. Side effects may include a sedated feeling, dizziness, vomiting, and sweating. The risk of rebound, dependency, and addiction exists.

Some examples of opioids are Percocet, Vicodin, and Demerol. (See "Calling on Superhero Medications," later in this chapter.)

Stopping Migraines Upfront: Prophylactics

During your info-gathering venture, you may become intrigued by the drugs called prophylactics, because they hold the enchanting lure of keeping migraines at bay entirely. Typically, if you tried avoiding triggers and using relaxation techniques and biofeedback, and you still can't control your migraines, your doctor may think that you can benefit from a regimen of preventive medications.

You're a good candidate for prophylactic therapy if you

- ✔ Have frequent migraine attacks (two or three a month), and they're so annoying that your quality of life is compromised.

- ✔ Have severe migraines that aren't relieved by forms of symptomatic treatment (treatment to relieve symptoms such as pain and nausea).

- ✔ Have menstrual migraine attacks that haven't responded to other methods of treatment. (A woman may be able to prevent migraine attacks by taking an NSAID a few days before starting her period, or during the first few days of menstruation.)

If your doctor thinks that preventive therapy is a good option for you, the goals are: less frequent headaches, less severe migraines, and improved quality of life.

But there are a number of reasons that you don't just jump willy-nilly into using preventives instead of trying to stop a migraine that has already begun. Check out the following downsides of prophylactics:

- ✔ **You need to be monitored.** Your prophylactic treatment has to be monitored by a physician, because each preventive medication has potentially dangerous side effects.

- ✔ **You're subject to side effects.** To reap the benefit (warding off headaches), you have to accept the possibility of living with side effects such as weight gain, hair loss, and so on. (See the descriptions of individual drugs in this section for specifics on side effects.)

- ✔ **You have to stick to a scheduled regimen.** This medicine won't relieve headache pain, so you have to take it every day to prevent a headache. Some people don't want to take drugs on a daily basis. Plus, prophylactic therapy just isn't necessary for those who only have occasional migraines.

Your doctor will usually start you on a low-dose migraine preventive and then gradually increase the dosage until it works well for you. Or he'll stop increasing the dosage if you find that the side effects become too annoying or you have reached the highest safe dosage. Don't give up on a drug and switch to another just because the low-dose version fails to help.

Some people find that prophylactics are very successful in preventing migraine attacks, while others find that they get less of an effect from the drug.

Prophylactics won't help a migraine already in progress.

Make sure that you follow a very specific doctor-prescribed schedule when taking prophylactics. Doing so will help prevent the spiral that starts a migraine. Along with taking the preventive properly, you should also eat a healthy diet, get enough rest, and exercise regularly to maximize the benefits of the drug.

The following sections cover some common groups of prophylactic migraine drugs.

Antidepressants

Some antidepressants, which are actually meant for treating depression, have crossover appeal because they can also be used to help prevent migraines. Possible side effects include constipation, dry mouth, anxiety, elevated blood pressure, and weight gain. Some examples of antidepressants are Elavil and Pamelor.

Elavil (amitriptyline)

This tricylic antidepressant is commonly used to treat depression, eating disorders, and chronic pain.

- **Modes of delivery:** Tablet, injection.

- **Possible side effects:** Sleepiness, dry mouth, constipation, weight gain, irregular heartbeat, impotence, nausea, and black tongue. Too much Elavil may cause convulsions, very low blood pressure, confusion, heart problems, or coma.

- **Don't take if:** You have hyperthyroidism, a history of seizures, liver problems, an enlarged prostate, glaucoma, you've had a heart attack recently, you've taken MAOIs within the previous two weeks, or you're pregnant or breastfeeding.

- **Doesn't interact well with:** Alcohol, barbiturates, carbamazepine, phenytoin, anticholineregics, guanethidine, and multiple other medications, so check with your doctor.

Pamelor (nortriptyline)

Pamelor, a tricyclic antidepressant, is most commonly used to treat depression and chronic pain.

- **Modes of delivery:** Capsule, liquid.

- **Possible side effects:** Dry mouth, sedation, weight gain, irregular heartbeat, nausea, black tongue, breast enlargement, loss of appetite, and ringing in the ears.

- **Don't take if:** You have an enlarged prostate, hyperthyroidism, liver impairment, heart disease, glaucoma, you're pregnant or breastfeeding, or you've taken MAOIs within the previous two weeks.

- **Doesn't interact well with:** Mixing Pamelor with MAOIs can be fatal. Nortriptyline can affect your reaction to alcohol. Pamelor can also interact with multiple other medications, so be sure to stay in close contact with your doctor.

Antiseizure medications

Some medicines aimed at seizure prevention are also good for migraine prevention. Possible side effects include hair loss, nausea, and weight gain or weight loss (depending on the medication). Some examples of antiseizure medications are Depakote, Neurontin, and Topamax.

Depakote (divalproex sodium)

Long used as an anticonvulsant, Depakote is also a successful migraine preventive. Some doctors use Depakote first when dealing with a migraineur who has seizures or certain psychiatric problems. Depakote won't help a migraine that is already under way.

✔ **Mode of delivery:** Tablet.

✔ **Possible side effects:** Weight gain, nausea, tremors, vomiting, hair loss, malaise, weakness, facial edema, anorexia, drowsiness, and liver toxicity. Stop using Depakote and contact your doctor if bleeding, bruising, or a coagulation problem occurs.

✔ **Don't take if:** You have liver disease or you're pregnant or breastfeeding. Too much Depakote may cause a drugged feeling or coma.

✔ **Doesn't interact well with:** Blood thinners (warfarin), aspirin, oral contraceptives, barbiturates, erythromycin, rifampin, diazepam, and zidovudine. Depakote interacts with other seizure medications, as well as multiple other medications, so check with your doctor.

Your doctor will monitor the level of Depakote in your blood.

Ergot derivatives

Ergot derivatives are drugs that reduce inflammation and help blood vessels constrict, thus relieving headache pain. Ergot derivatives aren't popular for migraine treatment, because they can't be used if you have high blood pressure, heart disease, or certain vascular diseases.

If you take ergotamine and experience numbness, tingling, muscle cramps, or coldness in your toes or fingers, call your doctor immediately.

Sansert (methysergide)

A derivative of ergot, this synthetic drug is similar to ergotamine meds. Sansert is used for migraine prevention, especially in people who experience disabling pain, but it's a last-resort migraine medication because it can have serious side effects.

✔ **Mode of delivery:** Tablet.

✔ **Possible side effects:** Nausea, vomiting, abdominal pain, weight gain, hair loss, insomnia, sleepiness, leg cramps, and, rarely, a serious condition that involves thickening of the tissue around the heart, lungs, or kidneys.

✔ **Don't take if:** You have heart or vascular disease, high blood pressure, thrombophlebitis, collagen vascular disease, or you're pregnant or breastfeeding.

✔ **Doesn't interact well with:** Imitrex and some other drugs (check with your doctor).

Don't suddenly stop taking this medication: You must be weaned over several weeks to avoid a withdrawal headache.

Beta blockers

The beta blockers, known for treating heart problems and high blood pressure, have proven to be crossover successes in the migraine-fighting arena. They help prevent migraines by relaxing blood vessels. Possible side effects include depression, fatigue, and dizziness. Some examples of beta blockers are Inderal, Blocadren, Corgard, Tenormin, and Lopressor.

Blocadren (timolol)

Blocadren is a beta blocker that has been approved by the FDA for the treatment of migraines.

- **Mode of delivery:** Tablet.

- **Possible side effects:** Fatigue, breathing problems, cold extremities, dizziness, slow heart rate, and chest pain.

- **Don't take if:** You have asthma or other lung problems, a slow heart rate, heart block (electrical disturbance in the heart), overt heart failure, heart or lung disease, low blood pressure, diabetes, hyperthyroidism, liver or kidney problems, lupus, or you're pregnant or breastfeeding.

- **Doesn't interact well with:** NSAIDs (the effectiveness of Blocadren will be reduced), ergot medications, calcium channel blockers, digitalis, quinidine, and other medications, so consult your doctor.

Inderal (propranolol) and Inderal LA (long-acting)

Inderal, which is often used for treating angina and high blood pressure, is a popular migraine prophylactic. This drug requires careful monitoring by your physician.

- **Mode of delivery:** Tablet.

- **Possible side effects:** Fatigue, sleep disturbances, insomnia, breathing problems, low blood pressure, slow heart rate, dizziness, cold extremities, impotence, and depression. Too much Inderal may cause an irregular heartbeat or seizures.

- **Don't take if:** You have asthma, slow heartbeat, heart block, or overt heart failure.

  Your doctor will consider whether there's a better medication for you if you're pregnant or breastfeeding, or if you have any of the following conditions: diabetes, hyperthyroidism, liver or kidney dysfunction, Wolff-Parkinson-White syndrome, lupus, or lung problems.

- **Doesn't interact well with:** Ergots, alcohol, other blood pressure medicines, antithyroid drugs, chlorpromazine, calcium channel blockers, theophylline, digitalis, haloperidol, cimetidine, plus many other medications, so check with your doctor.

Avoid stopping Inderal or Blocadren abruptly. Do not use either one longer than six weeks if it doesn't help prevent migraines.

Nonsteroidal anti-inflammatory drugs (NSAIDs)

Nonsteroidal anti-inflammatory drugs (NSAIDs) are used for abortive and prophylactic treatment of migraines. See the entry for Naprosyn under "Fighting Back: Abortive Medications for Migraines Underway," earlier in this chapter.

Monoamine oxidase inhibitors (MAO inhibitors or MAOIs)

Normally used for treating depression, the MAO inhibitors can also be used to prevent migraines. They're occasionally prescribed for migraine prophylaxis. Possible side effects include constipation, dry mouth, weight gain, and insomnia. The downside of these medications is their many negative interactions with certain foods and drugs.

Nardil (phenelzine sulfate)

This MAOI is used as a migraine preventive, but it's not used as much as other preventive medications, because it has so many possible interactions with drugs and foods. Typically, Nardil is used for the treatment of depression. In most cases, the drug's benefits are believed to be cancelled out by the risks (it can be fatal if you take it with certain other medications or certain foods!). Ask your doctor about side effects, medication interactions, and so on.

Calcium channel blockers

Calcium channel blockers, which were originally intended to treat high blood pressure and heart disorders, have been used to treat migraines with only mediocre success. They serve to interfere with calcium's ability to constrict blood vessels. Possible side effects include fluid retention, congestive heart failure, shortness of breath, and impotence. Some examples of calcium channel blockers are Isoptin, Verelan PM, and Calan.

Calan (verapamil)

Calan is a migraine-preventive calcium channel blocker. Verapamil is also marketed as Calan SR, Covera-HS, Verelan PM, and Isoptin. It is usually used to treat high blood pressure and angina. Some doctors consider Calan to be the best calcium channel blocker for preventing migraines.

- ✔ **Modes of delivery:** Tablet, capsule.

- ✔ **Possible side effects:** Dizziness, heart failure, constipation, nausea, low blood pressure, and flushing. Too much Calan may cause a drop in blood pressure and serious heart problems.

- ✔ **Don't take if:** You have low blood pressure, heart failure, sick sinus syndrome, heart block, irregular heartbeat or other heart or circulatory problems, muscular dystrophy, liver or kidney disease, you're pregnant or breastfeeding, or if you've had a bad reaction to a calcium channel blocker.

- ✔ **Doesn't interact well with:** Beta blockers, alcohol, ACE inhibitors, Tagamet, and multiple other medications, so check with your doctor.

Trying Newer Treatments

Some surprises have been unveiled during the ongoing search for new and better migraine treatments. One was the migraine-pain-fighting benefit of Botox, a substance that's injected into facial muscles to smooth wrinkle-prone skin. Studies are now under way to discover if Botox's migraine-relief trait is an accurate perception.

Another surprise was seeing the epilepsy drug Topamax cross over into the realm of migraine painkilling and discovering that it also results in weight loss. This drug has now gained great popularity for chronic migraines and rebound migraines, and reports of weight loss as a side benefit of taking the pill for headaches are not uncommon.

Smoothing wrinkles and headaches with Botox

Botox has been touted in all forms of the media for its wrinkle-smoothing properties. You may have heard of the widespread popularity of Botox parties, where women gather to sip wine and get wrinkle-zapping injections. Now we see Botox spreading its magic into the realm of headaches.

Some doctors are using Botox to treat migraines, and the FDA is looking at the possibility of approving it for this use. Unfortunately, because Botox isn't yet FDA-approved for migraine treatment, insurance companies usually don't cover injections, which can be pricey (about $300–$500 per visit).

Basically, Botox (or botulism toxin type A) interferes with the transmission of nerve impulses that cause muscles to move, thus making it a godsend for people with eyelid muscle spasms. So, in addition to being good for treating headaches, Botox injections can temporarily eradicate or ease frown lines between your eyebrows, furrows on your forehead, and crow's-feet on the skin around the outside corners of your eyes.

Some doctors think that blocking muscle tension with Botox upsets the chain reaction that leads to a migraine. So far, early clinical trials on using Botox for headache prophylaxis look promising.

With wrinkle removal, the effect of Botox lasts only three to four months, and it also appears that's the length of time that a migraineur will see a reduction in headache intensity and frequency.

Although botulism toxin type A can cause food poisoning when ingested, the Botox that is now being used cosmetically, as well as for treating migraines, is a highly purified and diluted form of the toxin that is believed to be safe in tiny doses delivered by direct injection.

Losing migraines and pounds with one pill

The new kid on the block for migraine treatment is Topamax, a prophylactic medication that has the surprising side effect of making you lose weight. Topamax is new to pain management, but the FDA approved it long ago to help control seizures in those who suffer from epilepsy. One study has shown that this drug (topiramate) reduces the occurrence and duration of migraines.

Doctors realized that this epilepsy drug had weight loss as a side effect when patients taking the drug began to shed pounds and have decreases in appetite during the seizure studies. Therefore, doctors weren't surprised when people began to lose weight after starting on the medication for migraine prevention. One woman lost 70 pounds in six months. However, most people who use Topamax for headaches lose 5 to 10 pounds.

Naturally, interest in Topamax has been high ever since Americans discovered that this migraine medication came with the appealing side effect of no-sweat weight loss. Today, this drug is touted as an excellent medication for helping to prevent migraine pain. Some women find that menstrual migraines are quite responsive to the pain-relief effect of Topamax.

If the dose of Topamax is increased too rapidly or used at a high dose, you may experience fuzzy thinking or develop kidney stones. Drink plenty of water!

Choosing a Delivery Method

Migraine remedies are available in tablets, wafers that dissolve on the tongue, capsules, shots, nasal sprays, and suppositories. Your choice of delivery mode will depend on these factors:

✔ **Nausea/vomiting:** You probably need a shot or suppository if you're worried about keeping a pill down. (You won't get any help from a pain-relief tablet that you upchuck!)

✔ **Urgency:** If you're having a horrible headache, and you go to the emergency room for evaluation and treatment, you'll probably receive an injection or intravenous medication if the doctor determines that you're having migraine pain. This delivery mode is used in such cases because you get pain relief fast (the medication takes effect quickly when injected or delivered by IV).

And, no, you can't go in for a once-a-month migraine preventive shot, but you can self-inject Imitrex (see the "Imitrex (sumatriptan)" section earlier in the chapter) when you're getting a headache.

✔ **Personal preference:** The type of delivery mode that works for you aesthetically is also a factor. Some folks hate capsules. Some can't stand suppositories. Others like wafers.

Calling on Superhero Medications

Sometimes you have to bring out the big guns when you're fighting a migraine.

Superhero medications usually work well, but they have the downside of putting you out of commission, as they sedate you in addition to killing your pain. However, if you're suffering from a horrible headache, you may welcome sedation (or perhaps even a couple of smacks on the head) if you think that it will make you feel better.

Typically, if you're resorting to a superhero medication, you aren't too worried about whether you'll be articulate when doing a work presentation. Hampered by debilitating pain and vomiting attacks, you aren't even going to work. Work may not even be a distant consideration for the moment. The big issue of the day is simply ridding yourself of agony.

Getting heavy-duty pain relief

Heavy-duty pain-relief medications include opioid drugs, steroids, combination medicines that contain butalbital, and the injectable NSAID Toradol.

Opioid drugs (narcotic pain relievers) are used to knock out very resistant headaches, but they can make your nausea worse, and they'll definitely make you feel too drowsy to function normally. They also have the huge downside of carrying the risk of addiction.

Pain relievers that contain an opioid are often injected; they provide rapid pain relief. Narcotic analgesics used to relieve migraines include Demerol (meperidine), Stadol (butorphanol), and Tylenol with codeine (which comes in a pill form).

NSAIDs

Over-the-counter NSAIDs such as Motrin and Aleve may work for minor-league head pain, but they usually won't do the job for severe migraines. Prescription Naprosyn often works for mild to moderate migraines. But for emergency situations, the superhero NSAID Toradol is a strong medication for tough pain problems.

Toradol (ketorolac)

Toradol works well for migraines that are moderate to severe. This drug is usually reserved for times when you fail to respond to other less potent meds. Toradol is used for migraines in the emergency room.

- **Modes of delivery:** Tablet, injection.

- **Possible side effects:** Nausea, dizziness, drowsiness, diarrhea, fluid retention, itching, and gastrointestinal bleeding and/or perforation.

- **Don't take if:** You have an allergy to aspirin or other NSAIDs, a history of peptic ulcers, a history of gastrointestinal bleeding or perforation, elevated potassium, low sodium, kidney failure, high risk of bleeding, or if you're breastfeeding. Also, don't take Toradol if you're taking aspirin, other NSAIDs, or probenecid. If you have liver or kidney problems or high blood pressure, or if you're elderly or pregnant, check with your doctor prior to taking Toradol.

- **Doesn't interact well with:** Toradol may affect the effectiveness of other drugs such as blood thinners, tranquilizers, certain antidepressants, diuretics, lithium, methotrexate, and ACE inhibitors (the blood pressure medications).

Opioids

Opioid drugs — narcotic pain relievers — can usually knock out headaches that are very resistant to treatment. When you're suffering with horrible head pain, that's very good news. Unfortunately, the price you pay for that pain relief can be threefold: extreme drowsiness, risk of addiction, and a worsening of your nausea.

Demerol (meperidine hydrochloride)

Demerol is used for severe migraine attacks or when you can't take other pain-relief medications.

- **Modes of delivery:** Injection, tablet, syrup.

- **Possible side effects:** Nausea, vomiting, sweating, drowsiness, constipation, and urine retention. Too much Demerol may lead to drug dependency, clammy skin, difficulty breathing, coma, seizures, and breathing problems.

- **Don't take if:** You have liver or kidney disease, thyroid problems, Addison's disease, irregular heartbeat, enlarged prostate, a history of seizures, a history of past or current drug abuse, or you're pregnant or breastfeeding.

- **Doesn't interact well with:** Tranquilizers, alcohol, antihistamines, certain antidepressants (the tricyclics), or MAOIs (when taken within two weeks of taking an MAOI).

Stadol NS (butorphanol)

Stadol is sometimes administered in an emergency room or doctor's office when a bad migraine fails to respond to other medications. You get quick pain relief, and the effects last for several hours. But, you can get addicted to this painkiller, and building up a tolerance and having rebound headaches are two other possible downsides of Stadol.

- **Modes of delivery:** Nasal spray, injection, intravenous.

- **Possible side effects:** Drowsiness, sweating, nausea, and high or low blood pressure. Also, addiction, rebound, and tolerance.

- **Don't take if:** You have lung, liver, or kidney problems, heart disease, problems with drug abuse, or you're pregnant or breastfeeding.

- **Doesn't interact well with:** Alcohol and sumatriptan nasal spray.

Corticosteroids

If you have prolonged migraine attacks, corticosteroids may be a good solution. Prednisone, for example, is very effective.

Deltasone (prednisone)

Although Deltasone is effective for treating migraines, it isn't often used, because it tends to have more side effects the longer you take it.

- **Mode of delivery:** Tablet.

- **Possible side effects:** Mood swings, insomnia, increased susceptibility to infection, ulcers, and high blood pressure. Prolonged usage may lead to weight gain, osteoporosis, and multiple other problems.

- **Don't take if:** You have a fungal infection throughout your body, or with a live vaccination, such as an oral polio vaccine. Your doctor may want to consider other treatments for you if you have problems such as tuberculosis, kidney problems, diabetes, cirrhosis, history of peptic ulcers, or if you're pregnant or breastfeeding.

✔ **Doesn't interact well with:** Barbiturates, rifampin.

If you take this drug, your doctor will need to monitor your progress carefully. Discuss with your doctor the dosage, side effects, drug interactions, and precautions.

Decadron (dexamethasone)

Decadron is used to stop migraine attacks that don't respond to any other treatment.

✔ **Modes of delivery:** Tablet, injection.

✔ **Possible side effects:** Mood swings, increased susceptibility to infection, ulcers, insomnia, and high blood pressure. Prolonged usage may lead to weight gain, osteoporosis, and multiple other problems.

✔ **Don't take if:** You have asthma, a recent heart attack, or a systemic fungal infection, or with a live vaccination. Your doctor may want to consider other treatments for you if you have problems such as tuberculosis, kidney problems, diabetes, cirrhosis, history of peptic ulcers, or if you're pregnant or breastfeeding.

✔ **Doesn't interact well with:** Barbiturates, rifampin, ephedrine, some diuretics.

Discuss with your doctor other aspects about this medication, such as dosage and other side effects.

Combination pain medications

Some of today's most effective and popular migraine drugs fall into the category called *combination pain medications.* These migraine drugs are so named because they contain acetaminophen or aspirin combined with another medication. The combo analgesics that contain a barbiturate or an opioid have habit-forming potential.

Fioricet/Fiorinal

Fioricet contains acetaminophen, butalbital, and caffeine. These three components are also found together under the brand names Esgic, Anolor 300, and Esgic-Plus. (Esgic-Plus has a lower recommended dose.) Fiorinal differs from Fioricet only in that it contains aspirin rather than acetaminophen. The medications that are combined in Fiorinal are also found together under the trade name Isollyl. Fiorinal also comes in a preparation called Fiorinal with codeine, which has the same components of Fiorinal in addition to codeine phosphate. These drugs are meant for occasional use in the treatment of moderate to severe migraines.

- ✔ **Mode of delivery:** Tablet.

- ✔ **Possible side effects:** Drowsiness, gas, abdominal pain, dizziness, drugged feeling, nausea, and vomiting. Too much Fioricet or Fiorinal may cause headaches, confusion, sweatiness, liver damage, breathing difficulty, coma, or a physical or mental dependency.

- ✔ **Don't take if:** You suffer from depression, current or past drug abuse, an allergy to any of the components of the medication, porphyria, peptic ulcers, kidney or liver impairment, suicidal tendencies, you're pregnant or breastfeeding, or if you're elderly and/or debilitated. Also, you should not use Fiorinal if you have an allergy to NSAIDs, bleeding or clotting disorders, gastritis, thyroid problems, an enlarged prostate, or asthma. Fiorinal should not be used by teens who have chicken pox or flu.

- ✔ **Doesn't interact well with:** Fioricet doesn't interact well with alcohol, antihistamines, MAOIs, muscle relaxants, tranquilizers, and narcotics. Fiorinal doesn't interact well with alcohol, beta blockers, MAOIs, blood thinners, NSAIDs, oral contraceptives, narcotic pain relievers, tranquilizers, and other medications, so check with your doctor. You shouldn't drink alcohol or drive when you're taking these drugs.

Bracing for the side effects of high-intensity medications

High-intensity medications usually do their job well — knocking out your headache — but you may also feel a bit disoriented and loopy.

If you're on one of the high-intensity migraine drugs, don't plan to operate heavy machinery, drive a car, or do anything else that requires hand-eye coordination and high alertness. You should also avoid making any serious decisions while taking these drugs. Plan on going to bed, letting the medication do its work, and falling asleep if you can. Hopefully, you'll wake up to find your migraine gone.

Getting Nausea Relief

The terminators for migraine-associated nausea and vomiting are usually administered through injection or rectal suppositories. The pill form will not be able to do the job if your body quickly rids itself of the helpful anti-nausea tablet.

When you take the *antiemetics* (medications that relieve nausea and vomiting), you get relief from nausea and vomiting, and a sedative effect that helps the pain go away. Some examples of a class of antiemetics called phenothiazines are Phenergan (promethazine), Compazine (prochlorperazine), and Thorazine (chlorpromazine). Some examples of other types of anti-nausea medications are Reglan (metoclopramide) and Tigan (trimethobenzamide).

The possible side effects of any of the antiemetics are drowsiness, involuntary movements, low blood pressure, and rashes. Migraineurs who use antiemetics typically experience few serious problems with the side effects.

Phenergan (promethazine)

Promethazine is an old favorite in the drug world. A well-known anti-nausea drug, Phenergan is usually administered in suppositories, which work well for people with nausea and vomiting because they can't keep pills down.

- ✔ **Modes of delivery:** Tablet, rectal suppository, syrup, intramuscular injection, intravenous.

- ✔ **Possible side effects:** Drowsiness, dry mouth, involuntary movements, dizziness, and blurred vision.

- ✔ **Don't take if:** You suffer from sleep apnea, asthma, enlarged prostate, glaucoma, a history of seizures, ulcers, heart disease, or if you're pregnant or breastfeeding. In addition, ill children should not take Phenergan.

- ✔ **Doesn't interact well with:** Alcohol and other medications that cause sedation.

Reglan (metoclopramide)

In some people, Reglan doesn't cause as much drowsiness as Phenergan or Compazine, so your doctor may prescribe it if you want to go to work or school with a migraine.

- ✔ **Modes of delivery:** Tablet, intramuscular injection, intravenous.

- ✔ **Possible side effects:** Drowsiness, involuntary movements, restlessness, dizziness, and depression.

- ✔ **Don't take if:** You have gastrointestinal problems, such as bleeding, obstruction, or perforation. Don't use with pheochromocytoma, epilepsy, and medications such as Haldol and the phenothiazines. If you have Parkinson's disease, a history of depression or breast cancer, or tardive dyskinesia, or you're pregnant or breastfeeding, talk to your doctor before taking this medication. Reglan is not recommended for children.

- ✔ **Doesn't interact well with:** MAOIs, alcohol, Bentyl, insulin, narcotics such as Percocet, and other medications, so check with your doctor.

Chapter 9

Sampling Alternative Remedies

*E*ven if you already tucked one or two mainstream pain relievers in your headache-bashing bag of tricks, it doesn't mean that you can't tack on a few alternatives to help spice up your treatment package. Of course, you need to check with your physician before trying any alternative remedies.

Some migraine sufferers find alternative approaches to be worth trying when first-line treatments fail. Other sufferers turn to these treatments for extra comfort during times of head pain. However, people who have severe migraines don't usually find relief via alternative treatments alone.

You can choose from a variety of alternative therapies, ranging from the bizarre (a visor-like device that massages your head) to ones that are known to offer significant relief for migraine sufferers (biofeedback).

When you try gimmicky alternative therapy products, such as the Relaxica Instant Tension Reliever that applies acupressure and massage action to soothe head muscles (www.reliefzone.com), you have little to lose but time and money, assuming the therapy is not invasive. At the same time, if you have any doubt about the item's safety or its compatibility with your other treatments, you should definitely check with your healthcare provider before going forward.

Relaxation techniques and biofeedback are two of the more successful therapies in the field of alternative migraine treatments, but they certainly aren't the only contenders vying for your attention. So if you like the idea of alternative therapies, check out the kaleidoscope of options in this chapter.

Don't let yourself be swayed into a buying a product just because it advertises itself as "all natural!" Advertisers can toss around the word "natural" freely, even if everything in the product is artificial. In other words, there are no standards, at least in the United States, regulating the use of the word.

Sampling Mind-Body Methods

For a moment, forget about medium- to hard-driving terminator prescription drugs and all those totally groovy over-the-counter meds. Now feast your eyes on the ultra-hip stuff — biofeedback and relaxation techniques, both of which, by the way, get an almost universal thumbs up from healthcare providers for their usefulness in treating migraines.

You may be able to relax away some of your pain or visually transport yourself to a pain-free state. In fact, these two techniques — relaxation and visualization (or guided imagery) — work extremely well for the treatment of migraines.

Calming techniques often used to relieve the pain of migraines include progressive muscle relaxation, deep breathing, meditation, and visualization.

Some alternatives, such as hypnosis and acupressure, come to you on shaky footing (especially if you're looking for your health insurance to cover your treatments). Because these options lack persuasive studies to underscore their usefulness in migraine relief, many healthcare providers consider them pretty iffy.

Some migraineurs believe that relaxation techniques and biofeedback help relieve their pain. Others argue that they produce little more than a *placebo effect* — it's effective only because you believe it will work. But the only way you can discover if these techniques have a pain-reducing effect on your headaches is to try them. And why not? They're certainly not going to hurt you, and they just may help.

Nevertheless, when you're looking for pain relief, the one treatment that you haven't tried yet may be the perfect fit for you.

Picturing yourself pain-free

Visualization (guided imagery) is a technique in which you dream up a special relaxation scene that you can mentally float away to, picturing yourself free from headache pain. You transport yourself to your own Shangri-La, where you finesse your headache pain down as many notches as possible. With a peaceful spot that you can visit anytime, you seek to relieve your migraines by visualizing yourself pain-free.

Your getaway scene must be one of your own choosing. You can select a video snippet in which you're rocking your toddler in your arms, lying on the beach in the sun, or sipping hot buttered rum by the fireplace. (Whatever makes you feel good.) The point is, you want to waft away to a place where you feel totally unwound and relaxed.

You may have to practice a bit to make this drill work, but when you do get it going, you can slip away anytime. In your private place, drink in peacefulness and subdue your migraine pain. Using visualization techniques may help you reduce the frequency of your migraines and alleviate the symptoms when a headache has already started.

When you perform visualization techniques, you persuade your brain to immerse your senses in your safe and soothing scene. You want to experience the smells, sights, and sounds of your relaxing environment. You practice using imagery to achieve relaxation during your headaches or when you feel them beginning.

Keeping your cool with relaxation techniques

You can use relaxation techniques to stave off headaches that result from an overdose of daily stress. When you're stressed, your breathing and heart rate become more rapid, causing the blood flow to your muscles to increase. A prolonged state of these physical changes can lead to a headache and sleep difficulties (see Chapter 14 for more on migraines and the sleep-habit link).

Using relaxation techniques, you can slow your heart and breathing rates and decrease your brain's sensitivity, which may help keep your headaches from developing.

You can add relaxation techniques to your migraine treatment arsenal simply by studying up on the processes in the following sections or using an instructional tape.

Making your muscles relax

With progressive muscle relaxation, you take yourself through a slow, thorough ritual of concentrating on toe-to-head muscle relaxation. You start at the tip of your toes, contracting and relaxing your muscles, and then work your way up, gradually tensing all your muscle groups.

Start by lying down with your arms at your sides, palms down. Make your hands into fists, tighten them, and then relax them. Imagine all of your muscles losing their tension and becoming pliable. Go through the tense-and-relax process with the following body parts, one by one: toes, feet, legs, pelvis, stomach, back, and shoulders. Tense for about 10 to 15 seconds, and then relax for 20 seconds.

Combining this practice with deep breathing can reduce migraine pain for some folks. You have to practice this technique, of course, to get good at doing it, and you must be able to place extreme focus and attention on each muscle group. In other words, if you tend to be very anxious, this exercise won't be your thing, because you'll find it hard to lie still long enough.

Meditating on meditation

Sit in a relaxed position, close your eyes, breathe deeply, and repeat a mantra to reach a state of relaxation. Your mantra can be something you choose or the often used meditation mantra "om."

A *mantra,* by the way, is a calming and pleasant word or sound that you repeat to increase your focus on the task at hand. You try to rid your mind of stress in order to achieve a peacefulness that may help your headache pain recede. If you don't want to utter mantra sounds, simply focus on your own breathing.

Free your mind to concentrate on easing yourself away from the pain of a migraine. Relax and let calmness caress you, but don't try too hard. It may take time to get the drift of meditating.

Think about creating a natural oasis from pressure.

Breathing deeply with deep breathing

Breathe deeply and slowly, and conjure up relaxing, positive images in your mind. Deep breathing serves as a strong foundation for relaxation. Use calming sentences to help you attain a state of peacefulness that will aid you in reaching a plateau of reduced pain.

To get started, place one hand on the lower part of your ribs, above your abdomen. Keep your hand in place and breathe deeply through your nose, letting your ribs expand and contract fully. After a couple of minutes of breathing in and out, exhale deliberately and fully through your mouth. Count to three as you let your stomach push the air out. After you exhale completely, inhale through your mouth for a count of three.

You should continue repeating the exercise for several minutes. You can practice this exercise when sitting or walking.

Harnessing the power of suggestion

Hypnosis is a trancelike condition in which subjects may be responsive (with certain limitations) to suggestions made by the person who places them in the hypnotic state. In the case of headaches, this state of heightened awareness and concentration may be used to manipulate your perception of pain.

A hypnotist can use the power of suggestion to relieve migraine pain as well as the symptoms of migraine, such as nausea and vomiting. The goal is to get to the mind's subconscious by inducing a relaxed and trancelike state. When your mind is in this state, you're open to receiving and embracing ideas that the hypnotist plants (or suggests). In the case of migraines, you look to substitute your negative thoughts on migraine development with positive thoughts.

If you want to find a good hypnotherapist, you can check the following Web sites:

- ✔ American Association of Professional Hypnotherapists, `www.aaph.org`
- ✔ National Board for Certified Clinical Hypnotherapists, `www.natboard.com` (click on "Consumer Info/Where to Find a Therapist")

Therapists routinely use hypnosis to treat everything imaginable — from substance abuse to chronic pain. The success rate of hypnosis varies. In some cases, it may be completely successful. In other cases, it may not work at all. You have to decide whether it's right for you.

Before you dismiss hypnosis as a little too out there, we want to banish one major myth: You are absolutely *not* under a spell when you're hypnotized. No, hypnotism is an interactive process between the hypnotist-therapist and you. And it's really not spooky at all. Some people like this type of therapy so much, that they choose to learn self-hypnosis.

You don't have to sing 'Billy Jean' to love oxygen

Songbird Michael Jackson has a "youth-maintaining" hyperbaric oxygen chamber (or so we've heard). You, too, may be able to benefit from a hyperbaric oxygen chamber. These chambers are thought to be effective in relieving the pain of cluster and migraine headaches. (No moonwalking or cosmetic surgery is required.) You can ask your headache specialist if this treatment is something you should try.

With hyperbaric oxygen therapy, you're put in a hyperbaric chamber where you breathe 100 percent oxygen at a pressure that is greater than that within the body tissues or fluids. Some hospitals offer this specialty treatment, but it's very pricey. A healthcare staffer must perform this treatment for you, making it much more costly than the at-home alternative therapies, so it's a somewhat impractical solution to relieving your migraines.

Your insurance probably won't cover hyperbaric oxygen therapy for the treatment of headaches. On the other hand, if you have money to burn, and hyperbaric oxygen therapy sounds fetching to you, you can ask your healthcare provider where the treatment is offered.

Note: One small trial showed extreme relief from the pain of acute migraine when hyperbaric oxygen was used. Some participants' severe headaches changed to mild or no pain after 40 minutes of treatment. The study looked at hyperbaric oxygen versus *normobaric oxygen* — breathing oxygen at normal pressures — for treating acute migraine, and results pointed to a large difference in favor of hyperbaric oxygen. (From "Evidence-Based Guidelines For Migraine Headache: Behavioral and Physical Treatments," by J. Keith Campbell, M.D.; Donald B. Penzien, Ph.D.; Eric M. Wall, M.D.; sponsored by the U.S. Headache Consortium.)

Hypnosis can be compared to trancelike states that everyone has experienced:

- You're driving, and you're mentally focusing on some problem or obsessing over something. Suddenly you find yourself pulling up to your destination. You're surprised when you realize that the only way you could have traversed your familiar route was by turning on your automatic pilot. This state of mind seems almost magical, and somewhat disconcerting.

- You're doing paperwork or computer work while watching television, but you're so into the project, that absolutely none of the TV sound really permeates your mind. It's as though the TV has been muted.

Entertaining positive thoughts on a regular basis can make your immune system work better, reduce pain and anxiety, and enhance your health.

For some migraine sufferers, hypnotherapy is a truly effective way to curb pain. For others, the positive impact of hypnotherapy stems from having a feeling of being in control. This uplifting feeling can help migraineurs find relief.

Many migraineurs find that having some control over the migraine force can be extremely empowering. This, in turn, may lead to an enhanced ability to reduce your own headache pain.

Some people seek migraine relief by having a therapist hypnotize them, while others use self-hypnosis.

Being hypnotized by a therapist

If you go to a hypnotherapist for migraine relief, you can expect to be moved into a state of trance by listening to a therapist's velvet voice telling you how heavy your eyelids are getting or how relaxed you are, or something similar. You may be told to count backward and fall ever more deeply into a state of relaxation.

The therapist offers positive suggestions that are meant to ease your pain. You should brush away any extraneous thoughts that get in the way of these soothing suggestions.

Here are some positive affirmations that you may want to try:

- "I'm going to awake feeling relaxed and unworried, free of headache pain."

- "I do not want to hurt; I do not want to lose valuable time because my head is hurting."

- "I am empowered to banish my pain."

- "I'm imagining that my skull is bound by a headband that is too tight, so I will simply unwind it, remove the headband, and free myself from the throbbing pain. When I do this, the ache will be gone, and I can use this same approach again if the pain comes back."

To bring you back out of your hypnotic state, your therapist will plant a few last thoughts as to how you'll feel when you return to a fully conscious state. Your therapist wants you to experience a pain-free, relaxed state of improved health and empowerment — your migraine pain is diminished, and you're back in action.

Empowering yourself with do-it-yourself hypnosis

You may be able to perform self-hypnosis after watching videos or listening to audiotapes. You're more likely to have success with self-hypnosis, though, if you take lessons from someone who has credentials in hypnotherapy.

With self-hypnosis, you can calm and lead yourself into deep relaxation. Using music or the repetition of a soft sound, you reduce the noise in your head by replacing it with relaxing, stress-curbing thoughts. You get loose and comfy, and focus on ridding your body of tenseness. You may use a special calming scene (such as a secluded room) as a retreat for your do-it-yourself hypnosis spot. Breathe slowly and deeply, and repeat your mantra. In the trance state, you may want to listen to a tape that has positive messages. (You can find tapes that speak about how you're banishing the headache pain, sending it away.) When negative thoughts fly into your brain, you should wave them aside.

Gradually, via self-hypnosis, you may be able to reduce the distress that is attached to your migraine pain. As you lower this distress somewhat, the pain eases.

To release yourself from the hypnotic place, you count backwards from ten to zero, and in so doing, you reassure yourself — "I'll feel calm, pain-free, and content upon awakening."

For more information on self-hypnosis, check out the Psychological Self-Help Web site at www.mentalhelp.net/psyhelp.

Using autogenic training

Autogenic training refers to a technique used for achieving relaxation based on concentration and an awareness of sensations. With autogenic training, the power of suggestion is called upon to decrease muscle tension and increase the flow of blood. During self-hypnosis, you transport yourself to a calm state by mentally focusing on the individual parts of your body, imagining each as warm and heavy to counter the usual migraine sensations.

Get good at this practice, and you may be able to decrease headache pain or, in some cases, keep it away altogether. Autogenic training is basically an exercise of mind over matter when dealing with your migraine pain.

Banking on biofeedback

Both children and adults sometimes benefit from biofeedback as a treatment for migraine (and tension-type) headaches. Biofeedback is painless and effective. It works best when used on a regular basis.

In the context of migraine treatment, *biofeedback* is a technique in which you're taught to relieve migraine pain by manipulating your own physical signals. Researchers have found that people can alter their involuntary responses when they're fed back information about what's happening in their bodies, whether that information is transferred visually or audibly. Some of the functions that are measured to provide feedback are heart rate, sweat gland activity, brainwave activity, skin temperature, and muscle tension.

For example, flashing lights or beeps may be used to indicate that your muscles are tensing up. You can slow down the flashing or beeping by relaxing your muscles. Eventually, you learn to perform the response even when you're not hooked up to machine sensors. Some of the problems that biofeedback can be used to treat are migraine and tension-type headaches, premenstrual syndrome, incontinence, panic and anxiety disorders, high blood pressure, bedwetting, and Raynaud's disease. Performance enhancement in athletes is another use for biofeedback.

Biofeedback teaches you to control your body's responses with concentration. During the procedure, a machine feeds back information via instrumentation (versus an inborn biological loop in your body). As the machine tells you how you're doing, you can learn to raise and lower your body temperature levels and promote relaxation. Regulating the temperature of the hands and feet (migraineurs often have cold extremities) allows some migraine sufferers to reduce the number and intensity of their migraines.

If you're interested in trying biofeedback, consult with a certified biofeedback practitioner who specializes in migraines. You can find one through the Biofeedback Certification Institute of America Web site at www.bcia.org.

Working with Behavioral Headache Bashers

Behavioral therapy focuses on the role that behaviors play in migraine progression. You find out how you react when the pain starts — or when you feel a headache coming. Then you sample new-and-improved ways of reacting and see if they ward off pain.

You won't know if a new behavior can really affect your migraine until you sample it — although, you have little to lose by giving new behaviors a try.

With behavioral therapy, you and your doctor or therapist will

✔ **Set up the problem to be resolved.** You want to iron out your sleeping problems so that they no longer trigger migraines.

✔ **Establish a goal.** You want to get restful, healthy sleep (of about the same duration) nightly.

✔ **Monitor your progress.** You want to determine if the methods being used to alter your sleep-preventing behaviors are working.

✔ **Modify environmental factors that are contributing to your sleep problem.** You want to create a sleep environment free of distractions, lights, and noises that can interfere with your slumber.

✔ **Begin using behavioral therapies.** You may use reframing, self-talk, desensitization, role-playing, and positive thinking.

You can try behavioral changes alone or in conjunction with drug therapy. (Seek the advice of your physician.) Basically, you're going to replace unproductive behaviors with ones that actually help you manage your headache pain or keep it from forming.

The following tips will help you replace unproductive behaviors with migraine-curbing habits:

✔ **Try simple methods first:** Try to manage your pain with simple behaviors (walking, neck massage, breathing and relaxation techniques) instead of reaching for pain-relief medication at the first twinge of a headache. (This rule applies only to people who have mild to moderate migraines. If you have severe headaches, you need to take something at the onset of your headache, or you'll end up suffering for sure.)

✔ **Check your support network:** Assess your response to having family members baby you when you're feeling bad. Is this a strong positive, a neutral, or a negative? If you experience a great deal of gratification when you're given extra attention, your behavioral response may be a subconscious factor in prolonging your migraine symptoms. Why not ask the coddling family member to do a little less sympathizing during your next headache episode so that you can see how her behavior affects you?

✔ **Save the meds for last:** Redefine the phrase "take as needed for pain." Reward yourself in some way when you're able to resist the positive reinforcement of a pill that at least takes the edge off the discomfort. See what happens when you try living with a dull ache — you can see if the headache goes away with rest and relaxation.

Again, this recommendation doesn't apply to migraineurs who experience severe headaches. If you have severe headaches, your challenge is to continually monitor your intake of pain meds so that you don't become disabled by a dependence on pain killers.

✔ **Wage war on negative self-talk:** When you think "Why me?" or "Bummer, my head's killing me — I never get to go anywhere!" replace the thought with a matter-of-fact "I'll feel better soon!" or "This is a family legacy I must live with, along with the many good traits I inherited."

✔ **Own your migraine fate:** Reframe your headache issue so that you think of yourself as the person in charge of your migraines — not someone who is victimized by them.

Fighting pain with fitness

Assuming that you don't have trouble with exertion headaches (see Chapter 4), you can use movement to help ease the pain of your headaches. It will relax you and help decrease your stress.

You can expect to see a reduction in the frequency and severity of your migraines if you follow a consistent program of walking, cycling, swimming, or aerobics classes. Time and again, studies underscore the importance of consistent aerobic exercise for overall health maintenance and enhancement. (See Chapter 12 for more on exercise.)

Giving yourself a neck massage

Many of the people who suffer from migraines and tension-type headaches also experience a great deal of muscle tightness in their upper back and neck.

If you're a heavy-duty computer user, you're almost sure to have knots in your upper back and neck muscles from all the hours of sitting in a rigid position. Unraveling these muscle kinks may help to relieve your migraine pain.

Feel the base of your neck and your upper back for tight muscles. After you find them, press down with your fingers and give those knots a gentle but firm massage. Think of what you're doing as a way of softening the knots in your neck and back. Then use your fingers to massage your neck. Be sure to address your skull, temples, and ears. Be very gentle. Stop massaging occasionally to move your head up and down, and side to side. If you enjoy massage oils (and strong smells aren't headache triggers for you), rub them into your skin and savor five or ten minutes of soothing self-massage.

If your headache seems to get worse during a neck massage, or if the massage causes intense pain, stop immediately and see your doctor.

Finding belly laughs

Vote early, vote often. Laugh early, laugh often. And while you may end up regretting the candidate you choose, you'll absolutely never in a million years be sorry that you laughed.

In today's pressure-cooker society, few of us spend enough time doing the stress-reducer that's the best: the good old, hearty belly laugh. It's basic, free, and easy.

So, if you can't break into laughter whenever you feel like it (you're not Whoopi Goldberg or Bill Murray, after all), just call on some funny or silly resources. Start with that special someone who always makes you laugh. Spend some time with her, and you'll be cracking up in no time. These visits can be a good preventive for migraines, but after your head pain starts, they will be out of the question.

You can also watch a sitcom that never fails to tickle your funny bone, or turn on your DVD player and view one of your all-time favorite funny movies (some classic laughers are *Stripes, National Lampoon's Vacation,* and *There's Something About Mary*). Movies that you can listen to without giving your full attention (because you know all the punch lines already) are perfect for migraine days.

Read the comics (there's a reason they call them the funny pages) or a David Sedaris story; play with a baby or a baby animal — a kitten or puppy; ask a four-year-old to describe anything. For migraines, as for life, laughter truly is the best medicine.

Pursuing Alternative Physical Treatments

Physical treatments can be used to help prevent migraines. A number of approaches to physical treatment are available, including acupuncture and cervical (or neck) manipulation and mobilization therapy.

You may decide that you don't want acupuncture needles poking out of your body. Sounds like pure fright night, right? Similarly, your heart may not hum at the thought of being "cervically manipulated and mobilized."

You may want to try these physical treatments for the following reasons:

✔ You want to avoid using medications, or you don't do well on migraine drugs.

   If you're mainly trying to avoid drug therapy, don't kid yourself if you receive no real benefits from physical treatments. If you're still hurting big time, they're not working! Remember that drug therapy can be a safe alternative for getting rid of migraine pain. So you may end up at your pharmacy in the long run, anyway.

✔ You can't take migraine drugs because of other medical conditions.

✔ You're either pregnant or trying to get pregnant, or you're breastfeeding.

Balancing your energy with acupuncture and acupressure

Acupuncture has long been used for migraine treatment, and many people keep going back for more because it helps them. The treatment is based on the idea that your body has a harmonious flow of energy called *chi,* which is pronounced "chee." An acupuncturist seeks to restore your body to that state of balance by stimulating some of the hundreds of pressure points on your body.

To relieve pain and induce anesthesia, acupuncturists pierce the skin with fine needles. They can also use pressure — as in acupressure — heat, or an electric current. (The belief is that the stimulus serves to release pain-killing endorphins.)

It's still not certain how effective acupuncture is for treating pain, but it does appear to be helpful for some. If you decide to try acupuncture or another form of alternative treatment, keep track of how it works for you — you may even want to journal your results.

Manipulating your body to move out a migraine

Cervical manipulation is sometimes used as a treatment for migraines. It involves a therapist moving your neck beyond its normal range of movement. This method has its risks, including a remote chance of stroke. It should only be used as a last resort for headaches. Many experts think neck manipulation probably works better for tension headaches than for migraines.

Cervical mobilization involves the *oscillation* (or movement back and forth) of your neck within its normal range of movement. It is done to increase your neck's range of motion — it should be performed gently. Physical therapists and *chiropractors* (licensed professionals who manipulate body joints to restore normal nerve functioning) often perform both cervical manipulation and cervical mobilization.

Typically, a chiropractor or physical therapist looks for a structural (musculoskeletal) cause for your migraine. If she finds one, she will focus her treatment on the spot that is causing the migraine. She may zero in on a lack of mobility in a joint, a muscle spasm, or even bad posture. For example, if you have a muscle spasm in your neck, the therapist can mobilize and stretch the muscle to possibly reduce or eliminate your headache pain altogether. You may need several sessions of physical therapy, along with at-home exercises, before you notice any pain relief. For some people, it works. Others may get no relief from pain whatsoever.

Try massage before you turn to chiropractic treatment for migraines. Evidence suggests that the adjustments made by chiropractors are more helpful for lower back pain than for other conditions.

Chiropractors attend chiropractic college — not medical school — so they can't prescribe medication. Few physicians believe that chiropractic manipulation really helps severe migraines.

Micromanaging Your Own Treatment Program

You sit down with your headache specialist and come up with a plan. The doctor makes suggestions based on her experience and knowledge. You choose the treatments that will mesh smoothly with your life and ease your pain effectively.

Together you launch a first-round approach, which may or may not be the final word in your headache treatment plan. Some folks find answers in a matter of a few weeks, while others may pursue solutions for months. Either way, you're actively involved in the process — and the outcome.

Your treatment plan will feature the following elements:

- ✔ All of the treatments you're going to use
- ✔ A Plan B treatment for those times when Plan A doesn't give you pain relief

When your treatment plan is firmed up, be sure to share it with all concerned: your primary care doctor, headache specialist, and (if you have one) psychologist or psychiatrist.

Charting new migraine patterns after treatment changes

You'll hang on to some of the ideas in your treatment plan, and you'll toss the others.

Keep journaling the patterns of your migraines — frequency and severity, and triggers — every time you make treatment changes. With a journal, you'll be able to stay abreast of what is working and what isn't working, as well as what is making things worse.

You may want to keep a chart or headache calendar so that you can track the days you miss work or school (due to migraine), keeping notations on the treatments you use.

Marshalling the troops: Cyber-updates and support groups

Your treatment plan should be a living, growing thing. Sure, you may come up with a nice nucleus, but don't be afraid (with the help of your doctor) to add or embellish as the years go by and new therapies become available.

You can stay on top of what's happening in the world of migraine treatments via your doctor, the Internet, and support groups. The following Web sites provide migraine information and support:

- ✔ American Council for Headache Education: www.achenet.org
- ✔ American Headache Society: www.ahsnet.org
- ✔ Find Natural Treatment: www.migraines-findnaturaltreatment.com
- ✔ JAMA Migraine Information Center: www.ama-assn.org/special/migraine/migraine.htm
- ✔ National Headache Foundation: www.headaches.org
- ✔ The National Migraine Association: www.migraines.org
- ✔ World Headache Alliance: www.w-h-a.org

Migraine support groups include the following:

- ✔ Headache Area of Neurology WebForum: http://neuro-www.mgh.harvard.edu/forum/HeadacheMenu.html
- ✔ HealingWell.com Migraine Headache Community: http://community.healingwell.com
- ✔ HOPA HEADACHE HI-WAY: http://home.att.net/~headoffpain
- ✔ Migraine Support 4 Young Women: http://groups.yahoo.com/group/migraine_support_4young_women/

Consulting the Internet for health information can be quick and useful, but the information you find is not always correct. You should check with your healthcare provider before actually starting any new headache treatments. Be sure to discuss the safety and efficacy of the treatment, and whether it mixes well with your current treatments.

Chapter 10

Making Medical Decisions Even When You're Migraine-Hazy

Someone's asking questions, but your head hurts too much to answer. You can't think! You see the form of a doctor — you notice the white lab coat and the M.D. embroidered after his name. He's saying, "Do you understand that you may need a shot right now?"

The problem is, you're barely coherent. You have trouble making judgment calls when you're in the throes of a mind-bending, brain-blowing migraine. You're having a moment, all right — but not the good kind. Moments like this are the stuff legends are made of — very scary ones.

So, if you're a migraine sufferer, doesn't it make sense to plan ahead for just such a situation? You can design a game plan for what you will do when you get caught up in a bad headache cycle and you're barraged with questions. You can master certain survival tactics that you can draw on when you're feeling drawn and quartered. You can look objectively at the symptoms that can send you to the emergency room. You can line up a friend or relative to be on-call just in case you ever need to take a trip to the emergency room (and you're not able to drive).

Hopefully, you'll never need your migraine hazy-head plan. But there's a certain comfort in knowing that you have it.

Making Good Choices Despite the Migraine Haze

You're hazy from head pain, migraine meds, or both. Knowing what to do when it feels like a migraine has turned your mind to mush is a key part of migraine management. If you've already experienced this uncomfortable state, you know that making good decisions is one of your biggest concerns when you face a migraine fog.

During an incapacitating migraine, you have some vague notion that you're very sick and that other people — maybe doctors — want to know about the medications you've taken and the things you're allergic to. Unfortunately, you're in such a deep hole of pain, that coming up for air to answer these questions seems almost impossible.

You can do two things to improve this type of situation: Stick to non-mind-blurring medications and apply some survival techniques.

Using non-mind-blurring medications

The good news is that you may be able to avoid a medication-induced migraine haze altogether. The not-so-good news is that the non-mind-blurring medications you can take for pain are generally less effective than their stronger, more mind-altering cousins.

Over-the-counter medications such as acetaminophen and ibuprofen, and prescription drugs such as Midrin and Imitrex (which may cause drowsiness in some people) don't cause a migraine fog in most people.

If you find that the pain relievers you're currently taking lead to a level of incomprehension that makes you nervous, switch to a medication that's not as strong but is still effective at reducing the pain — or, if you're real lucky, knocking out the headache altogether.

Mastering survival skills

You can use certain survival skills to help you negotiate a blurry migraine fog. Maybe it's overkill. Maybe it's a migraineur's perfectionism. But some people like to set up an emergency-scenario game plan, just to feel covered in case the time comes when a headache takes them to the mat, rendering them incapable of handling a serious situation.

Using care when self-medicating

When it comes to negotiating a migraine brain-fugue, you don't want to make the mistake of gobbling down any and every pain medication in sight. You also want to avoid taking one type of pain-relief pill and, when it fails to help, immediately popping a few pills of another type of medication.

Jump off the self-medicating carousel and call your doctor if your headache pain is making you desperate or causing a lack of good (or rational) judgment. If necessary, get someone to take you to a healthcare provider.

If your headache is getting more severe, or your migraines are becoming more frequent, improvising on your migraine-management plan is probably the least effective way to help yourself. In these situations, you need to see a doctor.

Overmedicating may actually make you feel worse than your migraine ordinarily does. Check out Chapter 2 for a harrowing description of the rebound headaches that can last for days as a result of overmedicating. (Unfortunately, those days may feel like years.)

Designing a plan

Decide in advance (at a time when you're headache-free) what you're going to do when a migraine makes you feel out of it. You can refer to your plan when you begin to feel hazy from your migraine. Do anything you can to put a contingency plan in place that will help you rest easier, knowing that you're prepared *just in case.*

Here are some ideas to include in your emergency plan for dealing with a severe or abnormal headache:

- ✔ Call 911 if you live alone. Don't take a chance on driving if you suspect that you may be in dire straits.

   If you live with someone, brief that individual on what you're preparing for and what you would like for him to do if you think that you may have a dangerous headache (see Chapter 18 for more on dangerous headaches).

- ✔ Have a caring friend or relative (who lives nearby) on-call (see the following section).

- ✔ Brief a responsible party on your wishes in the event that you're rendered unable to make a decision regarding surgery or some other form of treatment. You may wish to sign a document that's called a *durable power-of-attorney for health care,* or a *medical directive.* (It's a good idea for older people to do this, anyway.)

   By signing a medical directive, you authorize the kind of treatment you prefer if you ever have an irreversible medical condition. The durable power of attorney for health care assigns decision-making to a relative or friend in the event that you become mentally incapacitated or unconscious. The assigned person has the right to sign checks, give medical consent, and make other arrangements. Durable power of attorney can begin when the patient wants it to go into effect, or when the ill person becomes incompetent. It takes two physicians to declare someone *incompetent* (no longer able to make informed decisions based on the information that's given to him).

It may be smart to have a migraine emergency kit that will be ready to go if you have to make a trip to the emergency room. If bright lights make you feel worse, have dark glasses or a hat ready to shield your face. If noises make you flinch during a migraine attack, put earplugs in your kit. If an instant cold pack gives you some pain relief when a headache is excruciating, tuck one in your kit.

Of course, just being in a migraine haze doesn't mean that you should automatically head for the ER. You may feel fairly hazy after taking any kind of painkiller. In this case, you have to avoid operating heavy machinery (cars!) and keep a low profile at home. If your brain is on the fritz, don't try going to work or participating in activities. Err on the side of caution. Just try to rest, and ask someone to fetch you food if you get hungry.

Appointing an on-call person for emergencies

Recruiting a friend or relative for a possible migraine emergency is harmless, and it hurts no one. (No one is out any time or money.) If you need to put your emergency plan into play, having one less decision to make can save you and your screaming head.

Brief your on-call person on what you want him to do if you call with an emergency. Keep his phone numbers handy, and feel secure in knowing that he's standing by, ready and willing to help. Ask your on-call person to let you know when he's taking a trip, so that you can appoint a fill-in.

You may want your on-call person to do the following tasks:

- ✔ Pick up a prescription that your doctor has called in.
- ✔ Take you to the ER and make sure that the doctor who treats you knows what pills you're taking and your medication allergies. (See "Knowing what to expect," later in this chapter.)
- ✔ Call anyone who needs to be notified, and let them know that you're in the emergency room (if you're taken there).
- ✔ Pick you up from the hospital after the doctor sees you (assuming the on-call person is unable to stay with you).
- ✔ Run errands (pick up kids or pets, or buy takeout food).

Having an on-call person doesn't make you a weirdo or a hypochondriac — it just shows that you're ultra-careful. And that's not a bad thing.

Negotiating the Emergency Room

When you go to the emergency room, don't expect red-carpet treatment. Typically, the medical professionals in an ER are exhausted. They'll likely put your migraine emergency far down on their priority list (where it may rightfully belong), unless you're very specific about your symptoms, and you let them assess the seriousness.

If you have headache symptoms that point to a potentially life-threatening condition (see Chapter 18), let the ER personnel know what's going on the minute you get there. And don't let them minimize your concerns as though you don't know what you're talking about ("Yes, I'm sure you have a bad headache, Mr. Dark, and the doctor will get to you in a few hours.") — insist that you know the red flags of trouble, and that you have them (if you indeed do)!

Knowing what to expect

No matter how bad you feel, you (or the person who took you to the emergency room) will have to provide a brief medical history several times when you're in the ER — at the minimum, for a nurse and doctor. They need to know the details of your current headache (when it started, where it's located, any accompanying symptoms, what medications you took that day, and so on).

Going to the ER with a worst-ever migraine

Buddy was having a bad migraine, so he took his date home. He then returned to his own house, where he went to bed. After an hour, he knew that it was time to go to the ER — his headache was getting worse despite the one dose of Imitrex he took for pain. Furthermore, his headache fit the *worst-ever* description that he had read about in a book.

"My head hurt so bad, I had my roommate take me to the ER, and a doctor gave me an injection to stop the pain. It was a hellacious headache, all right, but I was just relieved to know it wasn't a stroke."

The doctor reassured him that he had done the right thing in going to the ER for evaluation. "Red-flag symptoms should never be ignored — better to leave the diagnosing part to the doctors."

To prepare for the background health information that you will also be asked for, it may make sense to carry a list with you in your billfold or purse. Such a list should include:

- ✔ Your past and current medical problems
- ✔ What medications you're allergic to
- ✔ All the medicines you take on a regular basis (including supplements)

When the doctor evaluates you, he'll check your blood pressure and other vital signs, and do a physical exam to try to determine if further testing is necessary. If he decides that you have a migraine headache and nothing more ominous, he'll probably give you a medication via injection or IV to relieve the pain.

Handling ER attitude

Some people who have gone the emergency-room route for migraine treatment often complain about the experience: "The doctor and nurses acted like I was a great big drug addict, just there to sneak some drugs!"

Sure, you may feel outraged when someone in the emergency room gives you an attitude, but you must remember that people do indeed try to use the ER as a somewhat anonymous way to snag some powerful drugs. It happens often, and sometimes the culprits are successful. So no wonder ER staffers are leery!

Some members of the ER personnel may look at you with some suspicion or seem to question you incessantly, but their goal is to treat you safely. No one's trying to be mean or coldhearted. Drug abuse is a reality of today's society, so you may have to live with a few inconveniences when you're legitimately seeking help for your head pain.

Don't get mad when you're in the ER. Don't take anyone's vigilant screening attitude personally. And do be patient. Emergency rooms are usually busy whirlwind places. The people working in the ER want to perform their duties well (just like you at your job). These folks hope that their work helps the patients they're treating. Antagonizing you isn't the goal of ER personnel.

Part IV
Committing to Lifestyle Changes

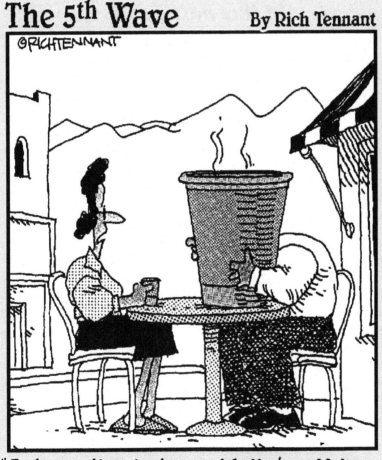

The 5th Wave   By Rich Tennant

"I know the doctor said that caffeine can help relieve your migraines, but don't you think you're overdoing it a bit?"

In this part . . .

This part shows you how to change your migraine-fostering habits — habits such as drinking red wine, snacking on junk food, late-night-partying, and anything else that puts your ultra-sensitive system on red alert and may lead to a debilitating migraine headache. Having the migraine tendency makes you a delicately calibrated instrument. Finding your headache triggers and steering clear of them can make an enormous difference in the number and severity of your headaches.

Part IV leads the way toward clearing your table of food culprits, changing your exercise from hurtful to helpful, and doing a fixer-upper on the headache-promoting aspects of your environment. It also explores the migraine/sleep-habit link and helps you pinpoint uneven slumber patterns and disorders that may be spurring your headache cycles.

Chapter 11

Catching and Rejecting Food Triggers

In This Chapter
▶ Pinpointing taste triggers that set off migraines
▶ Eliminating trigger foods from your diet

Some very ordinary foods can give migraineurs complete fits. So the sooner you key in on your own personal food triggers, the sooner you'll master migraine-sabotaging strategies.

Some studies (and migraine experts) don't support the belief that certain foods can be headache-provokers, but ask a migraineur who has experienced a direct correlation, and you may get a very different story.

And to make the matter full-tilt fuzzy, triggers aren't really the cause of your headaches. Genetics and chemical changes in your brain cause your headaches (see Chapter 4), but triggers still rate much focus and attention because they act as big players, initiating the series of cascading events that result in significant pain in a migraine-prone brain.

How aware of these food triggers do you have to be? Well, your goal in the food arena is the same as the one that applies to all other lifestyle variables: You're out to maintain your brain's delicate balance. Anytime you let a trigger sneak into the mix, the balance may get cockeyed, presenting the potential to spur a migraine.

Much of the information on migraine and diet is anecdotal and not based on strong science, but, at the same time, many people with migraines report that specific foods seem to contribute to their headache genesis. Therefore, they tend to make a habit of avoiding these foods. By keeping a headache journal (see Chapter 3), you can discover your own headache trends and figure out if any foods are triggers for you.

Essentially, you have to know your migraines, own your migraines, and take charge of your migraines. Only then will you figure out what's cool for you to eat — and what's likely to nudge those neurons into gnarly dysfunction when you sit down at the dinner table.

Tracking Down Dietary Triggers

You must track down and eliminate any dietary mischief-makers early in your migraine-busting plan. In fact, one of the most important steps in your entire quest for migraine answers is identifying food triggers.

A few foods and drinks are notorious for serving up headaches. These foods are listed in Table 11-1.

Table 11-1	Ingestible Potential Migraine Triggers
Meats	*Dairy (if lactase deficient)*
Aged, canned, cured, processed, or smoked meats	Aged cheeses
Bacon*	Buttermilk
Bologna*	Cream
Chicken livers	Ice cream
Canned ham*	Sour cream
Corned beef*	*Breads*
Fermented sausages	Freshly baked yeast breads
Herring, pickled or dried	Sourdough bread
Hot dogs*	*Vegetables*
Pâté	Broad beans
Pastrami*	Fava beans
Pepperoni*	Lentils
Salami*	Lima beans
Sausage*	Navy beans
Smoked fish*	Onions
Spiced meats	Peas
* contain nitrates, a migraine trigger	Sauerkraut

Fruits	Desserts
Avocados	Cake
Citrus fruits: Lemons, limes, oranges, tangerines	Candy
Figs	Chocolate
Condiments	Cookies
Olives	Snack cupcakes
Pickles	**Miscellaneous**
Salad dressing	Aspartame (an artificial, low-calorie sweetener)
Soy sauce	Beef concentrates
Seasonings	Cheese balls
Artificial sweeteners	Chinese food
MSG (monosodium glutamate)	Food dyes
Seasonings and spices	Meat tenderizer
Vinegar	Nuts
Beverages	Peanut butter
Alcoholic beverages (including wine)	
Caffeinated drinks	

Remember that food triggers are very individual. While lunch meats and nuts may be instant headache triggers for you, your sister (also a migraine sufferer) may be able to consume anything except red wine.

You can usually reduce your headache frequency by identifying your personal food and drink triggers and listing them in your migraine management plan up front. Some people are lucky enough to get rid of migraines completely by avoiding their dietary triggers.

Identifying migraine-inducing munchies

The tricky part of dealing with the food issue is this: Some triggers kick off headaches only when taken in certain amounts. Furthermore, dietary triggers don't contribute to headaches every time a migraine-prone person is exposed to them.

The names of some foods and additives keep coming up when migraine folks get together and compare notes. MSG (monosodium glutamate), red wine, and hot dogs have begun to rise to the top of the lists of tabletop items that appear to trigger migraines. While some experts dismiss the culpability of diet in migraine development, there will always be migraine sufferers who continue to dodge chocolate, lunch meats, and alcohol, no matter what the experts tell them.

Note that the following substances are the ones most often implicated as migraine triggers:

Checking additives, and chemicals, and preservatives (oh my!)

Aspartame, MSG, nitrites, and sulfites can all be headache triggers for some people.

Because many food triggers are actually caused by additives and preservatives, you may think that you can avoid these triggers by eating only natural foods. But you have to use common sense to identify which foods are natural, because food manufacturers are allowed to use the word "natural" pretty much any way they want when it comes to product packaging. So think of natural foods as foods that are grown or raised — vegetables, seeds, herbs, fruit, seafood, and meats. Natural foods aren't processed or packed with preservatives and chemicals, wrapped up in a box, and called "Your Magic-Meal-in-One Casserole." A long list of ingredients is usually a valid clue that the product isn't very natural. To ensure that your food isn't contaminated with antibiotics, pesticides, preservatives, or other unnatural substances, buy organic products, preferably locally grown.

- **Aspartame:** The artificial sweetener aspartame has two normal amino acids — aspartic acid and phenylalanine. Some researchers believe that an excessive intake of phenylalanine may increase the excitability of brain cells — this agitated state is associated with the chain of events in a migraine-prone brain that causes a pounding headache.

- **MSG (monosodium glutamate):** Monosodium glutamate is often used for flavoring and preserving foods. If you tend to have migraines, you may respond to the consumption of MSG with a fast and brutal headache. So be alert for the presence of MSG in your food. Read labels on the products you purchase. Look for some of MSG's many aliases, such as hydrolyzed vegetable or plant protein, yeast extract, sodium casseinate, autolyzed yeast, "broth," or "natural flavorings."

- **Nitrites/Nitrates:** When consumed, nitrites and nitrates can activate pain-sensitive nerves and trigger headaches in people who are sensitive to these chemicals.

  Nitrites are commonly used in bacon, ham, hot dogs, and other processed meats to preserve the meat's red coloring and prevent the growth of bacteria.

Nitrates and nitrites are part of the chemistry of plants. High nitrate levels are found in beets, radishes, and spinach.

Some heart medicines contain nitrates. We don't advocate eliminating medications if you try the elimination diet in the "Weeding out food triggers: The elimination diet" section, later in this chapter. Check with your doctor about switching to another kind of heart medication if the drug you currently take seems to trigger migraines.

Concern about the use of nitrites in foods was spurred when researchers noticed that nitrites could be converted into *nitrosamines,* chemicals believed to be carcinogenic in human beings. The researchers' findings led the USDA (United States Department of Agriculture) to place restrictions on the amount of nitrates and nitrites that are allowed in foods.

✔ **Sulfites (inorganic salts of sulfurous acid):** They have long been used to keep fruits and vegetables from turning brown, prevent black spots on shrimp and lobster, condition bread and pastry dough, and keep wine from developing bacterial growth during fermentation. Some supermarkets spray foods with sulfites to give them a fresher look.

Some common sulfite-containing foods are salad-bar items; soft drinks; maraschino cherries; French fries; trail mix; dehydrated, pre-cut, or peeled potatoes; molasses; soup mixes; hard cider; shrimp; condiments; baked goods; jams; canned vegetables and vegetable juice; pickled foods; gravy; dried fruit; potato chips; beer and wine; bottled lemon or lime juice; and tea.

On food labels, sulfites may also have the following names: sodium sulfite, sodium bisulfite, and sodium metabisulfite.

Provoking proteins: Amines

Some *amines* (compounds derived from ammonia) have been pinpointed as strong suspects in the lineup of headache triggers.

✔ **Tyramine:** This bully is found in the protein of foods. Levels of tyramine increase when foods are aged, fermented, or stored for a long time. High tyramine content is found in processed meats and cheeses, including brie, camembert, Roquefort, mozzarella, English stilton, blue cheese, sharp cheddar, Parmesan, and gorgonzola.

Tyramine is also the villain that makes red wine virtually the fastest migraine trigger in the Wild West — in other words, if you can't handle red wine, your head pain will be fast and brutal.

✔ **Phenylethylamine:** This nitrogen-containing compound is believed to be the key problem that triggers headaches in those who are sensitive to chocolate.

Reviewing regular foods

Some people report that common everyday foods such as veggies and nuts can trigger migraines. The reason that these foods cause problems for migraine-prone people is unclear, but there's no doubt that some pure, unadulterated or preserved foods are known migraine-raising culprits.

Jostling your beverage cart

If anything seems totally innocent, it's your beverage cart. But after you start sorting through your favorite drinks, checking for typical migraine triggers, you may be more than a little dismayed.

Well, there's always water. And you can have a glass of prune juice. (So, do you think the front-porch rocking chair can be far behind?)

Never mind — just keep your sense of humor and get real. You shouldn't have more than two cups of caffeinated tea, coffee, or cola per day whether you suffer from migraines or not. You must limit (or, ideally, cut out altogether) alcoholic beverages — especially red wine.

Don't forget that many drinks contain sugar substitutes such as aspartame. Many migraineurs report getting occasional headaches after consuming anything with this artificial sweetener.

Harping on alcohol

When migraineurs are asked to list dietary triggers, alcohol is always at the top of the list. Many migraine sufferers say that they just can't drink alcohol, especially red wine. On the other hand, some migraine sufferers can drink vodka, gin, and white wine without developing a headache.

Your brain gets such a going-over from the substances in alcohol that it should come as no surprise that the resulting reaction can make your head throb like crazy. Alcohol is such a potent trigger that many migraineurs report getting a splitting headache shortly after taking only a few sips of a drink.

If you keep drinking alcohol even though it's a trigger for you, be prepared to live with an entourage of alcohol hangers-on, including hangover migraines and headaches from the sulfites and tyramine in some beverages. In a word, alcohol is not your friend.

Coming upon caffeine's contradictions

Caffeine is the most schizophrenic of the food triggers. It can set a headache into motion, or it can cure one!

Caffeine is found in coffee seeds, cocoa, chocolate, and tea leaves. It's also found in most soft drinks and some pain relief medications.

For migraine folks, caffeine has major downsides. Your body becomes dependent on caffeine, so if you take in less than your normal amount one day (you usually drink three cups of coffee, and then you suddenly have just one), your body is going to rebel with a rebound headache (see Chapter 4). Also, it takes more and more caffeine to give you the stimulation you want. The upshot is that people tend to increase steadily their consumption of caffeine drinks.

Caffeine is a bugaboo: It can cause headaches when you curtail the amount you take in — whether purposefully (you're trying to cut down on the caffeine in your diet) or accidentally (*weekend migraines* come from drinking less coffee on weekends than weekdays). On the other hand, some migraine remedies contain caffeine as a therapeutic agent.

One woman with migraines says, "I got tired of having to make sure that every hotel [on trips] had room service or a coffee pot in the room. I knew that failing to get my morning fix would give me an awful migraine, so I began to view coffee as more of an enemy than a friend. I was hooked on the caffeine and didn't like the dependency." Interestingly, her caffeine intake started when she was a child and her parents gave her little just-for-fun cups of what they called "coffee milk" — a small amount of coffee diluted with lots of milk and sugar.

Assessing your water intake

Are you getting enough water? Or maybe too much? Water is the magic bullet that helps food fuel your body properly. Some people don't get enough water!

Proper hydration can be confusing — you don't want to drink so much water that you upset your electrolyte balance (which can lead to a very serious and sometimes fatal health situation), but you also don't want to drink so little that you get dehydrated, setting the stage for a headache and interfering with the smooth running of many of your body's processes.

Check out these recommendations for maintaining the proper intake of water:

- ✔ Drink eight to ten 8-ounce glasses of water per day. (If you need an incentive, drop a slice of orange, lime, or lemon in your water to spice it up.)

- ✔ Drink water before, during, and after physical activity; be sure to up your intake of water (above the eight to ten glass requirement) on days that you exercise.

- ✔ Make a special effort to drink water regularly while you're traveling by plane — plane travel tends to dehydrate you.

If you're on a weight-loss regimen that emphasizes low calories and increased water consumption, have a doctor monitor your progress so that your high intake of water doesn't result in a dangerous electrolyte imbalance.

TIP

Cooking without red wine or MSG

Red wine and MSG are the two most common migraine food triggers. If you're sensitive to either of these, you need to find recipes that don't use them. (Even if you don't have migraines, serving foods that contain red wine or MSG when you have guests isn't a good idea unless you know that no one suffers from migraines or has an allergic reaction.)

If a recipe calls for red wine, you can just omit the ingredient. You may want to add spices to compensate for the lost flavor.

Bear in mind that monosodium glutamate (MSG) is found in a number of seasonings and seasoning products, although it's best known as an ingredient in Chinese foods. MSG is used to pump up the taste of some processed meats, packaged foods, canned foods, meat tenderizers, seasoned salts, instant foods, TV dinners, roasted nuts, and potato chips.

The saying "you can't drink too much water" is inaccurate. Signs that your body may be over-hydrated include

- ✔ Confusion
- ✔ Dizziness
- ✔ Nausea
- ✔ Tiredness

Pulling the Plug on Migraine Foods

When you finally harness your dietary troublemakers, you'll feel like the Spider-Man of the headache world, cruising confidently along the erratic and skyscraper-filled metropolis of migraine-managing.

You may also try to control your reaction to any trigger that's impossible to eliminate. Perhaps you can tolerate a certain trigger if you eat it when other contributing factors aren't in place.

Facing the facts: Foods you love can be migraine triggers

"So," you may ask, "if avoiding a trigger is as easy as pinpointing troublemaking foods and drinks, how do so many migraine folks go wrong when it comes to diet?"

Well, facing the fact of dietary restrictions isn't easy. Some common traps that migraineurs fall into when trying to maintain a proper diet are listed here. See if you recognize your own downfall(s):

- ✔ **Deny, deny, deny.** For years, you may have suspected that certain foods aggravate your system and lead to headaches. But you love those foods! So you languished for a while in Denial Land, where you flat-out refused to believe that you couldn't eat Chinese food or that something as simple as diet soda could be a migraine-thug.

- ✔ **What, me worry?** And just because you're so delightfully human, you occasionally forget everything you ever learned about dietary precautions and turn into a freewheeling risk-taker who eats something "just this one time." When you hang out with friends, you probably yearn to come across as a sophisticated woman-of-the-world, and nothing seems less dignified than nerdily screening the foods you eat.

   Shortly thereafter, of course, comes the payoff — several hours of head pain and regret. You lie in a dark room and nurse yet another migraine, because your food trigger teamed up with some other troublesome factors, primed the pump, and set off your head pain.

- ✔ **Triggers are erratic and unreliable.** "But I love peanut butter, and it doesn't always give me a headache!" This phrase represents a common rebuttal from migraine sufferers. You're confused by the fact that one day a glass of red wine makes your head hurt like crazy, and then two weeks later you drink two glasses of wine and have no problem. Triggers are inconsistent. They sprout a headache only when they inadvertently team up with other lifestyle factor(s) that are problematic for you — such as intense exercise, stress, and hormonal ups and downs. You may not ever find a food that your body reacts to in a consistent way because of the interplay of two key factors:

  - Your system: Triggers must contend with your nervous system's preset migraine startup threshold. If you have an inherited migraine tendency, you have a low threshold. It's important for you to understand your threshold level so that you can relegate food triggers to a minimal threat.

  - The bombardment factor: The more triggers that gang up and assault your brain's control center, the greater the chance they'll be able to act as a battering ram that beats down your defense door and lets in migraine symptoms. Put together a brightly lit room, a high-chaos day, and a peanut-butter sandwich, and the cumulative trigger onslaught scales your threshold wall like a gang of buff and burly hooligans. After they're inside, here come the fisticuffs in your skull.

- ✔ **Being painstaking is a pain.** Identifying triggers takes careful scrutiny — who has time for that? Besides making a list of obvious foods that incite headaches, you have to dig around to discover all the sneakier triggers that aren't as obvious.

You may find that your migraine tendency makes you supersensitive to certain substances in food, such as additives or preservatives. You need to steer clear of foods that contain those substances if you find out that they're headache instigators for you.

To warm to the idea of abandoning foods that you really like, you have to adopt a for-the-greater-good attitude. To do so, examine (and try to accept) the following ideas:

- ✔ You (as a migraine sufferer) have a very sensitive nervous system. Your system just happens to be ultra-reactive to certain substances — caffeine, MSG, nitrites, tyramine, and nicotine.

- ✔ Your delicate system needs structure in order to stay happy and balanced. To provide this structure, eat at regular times (so that your body gets nourishment when it's expecting it).

- ✔ You may have to keep a food journal for a few weeks in order to identify foods and drinks that lead to migraines and figure out how you're going to reduce their roles as mainstays of your diet. If you take the time to keep a journal now, you can bypass tons of wasted hours — the ones that result from being sidelined with massive headaches spawned by food triggers.

- ✔ Remember that your system works best when you provide it with untainted foods — foods free of preservatives, coloring, and so on. (In other words, natural foods contribute to overall health and make migraines less likely.)

True food allergies are more serious than a sensitivity to food triggers that may give you migraines. If your body is broadcasting "Bad news! I'm allergic to this food or drug," you'll get hit with symptoms quickly: hives (an itchy red skin rash that breaks out in spots), with or without swelling of your lips and/or difficulty breathing, rapid heartbeat, vomiting, headache, and, in severe cases, anaphylactic shock. If you think that you're having a food allergy reaction, have someone rush you to the emergency room of the nearest hospital. For hives alone, see your doctor as soon as possible. If you have hives with other symptoms, such as swelling around your mouth or difficulty breathing, go to the emergency room immediately.

Weeding out food triggers: The elimination diet

You may decide to junk the offending food triggers right up front in your migraine-busting mission. This is called an *elimination diet* or *elimination process*. It's a good idea to have medical supervision during this project. With an elimination diet, you check to see if the removal of certain foods from your dietary regimen eliminates or reduces the number of your headaches. You essentially become an expert on what foods trigger your migraines.

Elimination diets are very controversial. Many headache specialists think that elimination diets are ineffective and that any findings will be iffy at best.

If you decide to go the route of an elimination diet, get your doctor's advice and help in monitoring your diet. She's familiar with good nutrition and your health status, and she can help prevent you from becoming dehydrated or nutrient-deprived.

Although the chart of headache-trigger foods in Table 11-1 may look daunting at first glance, don't forget that your personal list of tricksters won't include every item. You may have a special sensitivity to only two or three of the foods — or it may take several to trigger your headaches.

Trigger foods are more likely to give you grief if you're stressed at the time you eat them (see Chapter 22).

The following elimination approach requires you to drop all possible triggers until you no longer have headaches. You can personalize your elimination diet by dropping only the foods you suspect are headache triggers.

1. **Eliminate all potential trigger foods (see Table 11-1).**

   You can still eat vegetables, brown rice, fish, chicken, and fresh fruits (except citrus fruits).

2. **Drink lots of water.**

3. **Stick with nothing but bland food for two to three weeks.**

   Make it the healthiest food you can get your mouth around.

   Make sure that your very good intentions don't take you on the rocky detour of a low-blood-sugar headache. Low blood sugar (hypoglycemia) can cause many symptoms, one of which is a headache. So, to avoid a drop in blood sugar level that can lead to a migraine, eat several times a day, get enough protein, and steer clear of high-sugar, high-fat foods. *Grazing* (eating small meals or snacks every three to four hours during your day) is the ideal. You should also avoid crash diets.

4. **Add the potential trigger foods back in, one by one.**

   Be good to yourself by starting with a favorite. Keep the amount small.

5. **As you reintroduce each food, spotlight the troublemaker(s).**

   You can sample citrus fruits, which may trigger headaches, in varying amounts to see what you can tolerate. These fruits are nutritious foods, so you don't want to drop them if you can handle them in moderation.

6. **Ban food and drink triggers from your diet.**

By tweaking your eating with this elimination approach, you can cut the frequency of your headaches by half or more.

Eliminating certain foods, not all foods

When you get on the food-trigger elimination bandwagon, you may not feel jolly about the process. So take a matter-of-fact approach — you're doing this for long-range happiness. If you wrangle your headaches into a position where they're manageable, you can spend much less of your life in an unproductive, slow-motion migraine haze.

A magazine editor we know tells of a misadventure that reminded her how closely she needed to monitor her food and drink intake. Her migraine-prone body was too finicky for her taste, but it's the only one she has! She had to work with it, not against it.

"I had planned my company's Christmas party, and had a great time, hiring a band, and choosing the right restaurant for the occasion. Sure, I was stressed, but mostly, I was excited that so many people turned out. Suddenly, while standing there talking to someone, I felt dizzy and lightheaded. I'd never fainted, but I could tell that was coming. I melted into a chair and asked a co-worker to get me some Sprite or food. I'd been on a bland diet for weeks because I was trying to get rid of foods that were possible migraine triggers. I wasn't eating much, and on that particular day, I had a bowl of oatmeal for breakfast, a Diet Coke at lunch, and nothing else." As it turned out, she didn't faint, but she did end her festive evening with a bad migraine headache.

You may find it hard to own up to the truth of your eating situation — that having a headache tendency means monitoring what you eat and drink throughout your life. But if you can accept this hard truth, self-surveillance becomes an unconscious habit and not a daily nuisance.

You may feel like you're gearing up to eat — guess what? — absolutely nothing! But that's not the case, really. You just need to be realistic about what works for you — and what works against you (and spurs a headache).

If eliminating all possible food triggers seems too harsh, you can try giving up one possible trigger at a time. This approach takes longer, but it's less painful to go through.

If you're only going to try eliminating a few items initially, include the trigger foods and drinks that most commonly give headache sufferers trouble: alcohol (especially red wine), nuts, cheeses, chocolate, soy sauce, meat tenderizer, pizza, hot dogs, sourdough bread, avocados, and foods containing MSG or red wine.

You'll find your triggers during the elimination process, but you may also have to suffer through the withdrawal of giving up smoking and drinking alcohol and caffeinated beverages (if those indulgences are part of your current repertoire). Talk to your doctor about ways to handle the cold-turkey terror you may experience. Ask for support for any headaches you have.

If you drink alcohol daily (or almost daily), talk to your doctor before you quit, because you may need help getting through the process. The sudden cessation of alcohol can result in serious problems.

Chapter 12

Getting Physical with Your Migraines

In This Chapter

▶ Easing head pain with exercise

▶ Using body massage and physical therapy for migraine pain

▶ Knowing which forms of exercise to avoid

*E*xercise is good for your health and general sense of well-being. Massage and physical therapy make you feel great, also. But can these treatments give you good results for migraine pain relief?

In truth, exercise, massage, and physical therapy are just like many other migraine remedies. For some folks, they're assets. For others, they're not so helpful.

Loosening Migraine's Grip with Movement

Regular exercise can help you stave off headaches. It's important to discover what kind of exercise works for you, not against you. Some people have trouble with extremely intense workouts. At any rate, be sure to warm up before you exercise and be picky about the exercises you choose.

Basically, the benefits of exercise for your migraines are twofold:

✔ **It helps prevent migraines.** Exercise figures into migraine relief as a preventive. If you feel a headache developing, a brisk walk can sometimes stop the process.

✔ **It helps you handle headache pain better.** Exercise helps your body handle headache pain more effectively simply because it makes you a healthier person.

Regular exercise makes your body work more efficiently and calms your mind. Good exercise will almost undoubtedly reduce the frequency and severity of your migraines — and that's just one of the many payoffs.

Studies show that people who exercise regularly have better focus and quicker problem-solving abilities than those who don't. When you exercise, your brain chemistry is changed in a positive way, because exercise increases the production of *beta endorphins* (mood-boosting chemicals). Your mood is enhanced with higher levels of endorphins. This positive change helps prevent headaches, because part of what gets a migraine going involves chemical quirkiness in the brain — the endorphins help the brain stay stabilized.

Easing into exercise

If you suffer from migraines in general and exertion migraines in particular, you may want to slowly ease yourself into a new exercise program. You can do a long, slow warm-up and see if it keeps you from getting a headache. Or, if you can't handle high-intensity exercise no matter how much warming up you do, leave the high-impact exercise program behind and choose another form of spirit-lifting, heart-and-head-soothing movement — either active, such as low-impact exercise, or passive, such as massage or physical therapy.

Take a long, slow walk (15 to 20 minutes) before you climb on a bike or start an exercise class. Studies suggest that walking may help migraine sufferers acclimate their bodies to movement so that the vigorous exercise doesn't result in a headache.

Bottom line: If your workouts get to your head, warm up for a long time or try a calmer exercise program. But don't give up on exercise!

And if you're having trouble getting pain relief, chat with your doctor about the idea of trying passive therapies, such as different types of massage. Be sure to get his clearance before you venture into this new territory.

Sweating out migraines

If you're thinking about taking up some form of migraine-curbing exercise, consider these guidelines for picking a long-term program:

✔ **Get your doctor's clearance first.** Don't assume that your physical condition allows you to do just anything.

If you haven't exercised regularly for several months or more, have your physician check your heart, lungs, blood pressure, and other aspects of your health to evaluate your readiness for an exercise program. Health clubs, personal trainers, and fitness programs usually require clearance from a physician before they will let you start on a new regimen. You may also have to sign a waiver (health clubs don't want to get sued if you have a heart attack, slip and fall because you lack flexibility, or whatever).

If you have a history of not exercising, you can definitely benefit from having a qualified fitness consultant or personal trainer start up your exercise program (after you're evaluated by your doctor). A fitness pro can show you how to get maximum gain from your workouts. (One best-kept secret of all gyms is that many people don't get any benefits at all from exercising, because they don't use exercise machines correctly, they use poor form and execution, and/or they spend most of their time socializing.) The fee for an hour of personal training ranges from about $20 to $100, and you can typically get a startup regimen rolling in two or three sessions. The lower end of the price range ($20) is usually for a group session of two or three people.

✔ **Choose something you like.** You may have to sample several forms of exercise before you land on a winner. (Check out *Weight Training For Dummies, Yoga For Dummies, Power Yoga For Dummies, Mind-Body Fitness For Dummies,* and *Pilates For Dummies,* all from Wiley Publishing.)

✔ **Sign up for exercise that's convenient.** Join a health club that's close to home or work, or find a nearby park or high school track where you can walk. Studies show that people almost always abandon their workouts if they join a facility that is out of the way. People have a tendency to make excuses to avoid going to the club: "I need to start cooking dinner, and it's so far." "I forgot to take my workout clothes." "I hate driving all that way just to exercise!"

✔ **Do something that fits your nature.** If you're a group person, take a class. If you're a loner, you may find your niche in a solitary form of exercise, such as walking, running, or cycling.

To stay consistent with your migraine-fighting exercise program, give yourself pats on the back. When you're consistent with your exercise for three weeks, buy yourself a new pair of exercise shorts or a T-shirt. And tack up mental notes to remind yourself that your fitness routine is a huge plus for headache prevention and overall health — not a grueling duty that you have to slug your way through. Look at the process of sorting through possible types of exercise the same way you look at checking out a cool bookstore, a great vacation spot, or a wonderful new boutique. Consider exercise an adventure with very real payoffs.

To get the best results from your exercise, work on improving your diet. Try to get into a mindset that requires you to fuel up in a way that complements your fitness training. (This will fit well with your new and improved dietary plan for avoiding foods that trigger migraines — see Chapter 11.)

Keep your options open. Think of yourself as a freewheeling man- or woman-of-the-world who's cruising the Mall of the Exercise Universe, looking for something you like. The world of workouts is your oyster. Be picky. Be discriminating. Be realistic. You may find yourself doing something that ends up being the best hobby you ever had — and all because you were looking for a form of exercise that your migraines could chum up to!

Now check out some exercise options!

Combining weight training and walking

Walking and weight training are two low-impact (and helpful) forms of exercise for people with migraines. Neither is highly intense or known for spurring migraines. Although you can certainly choose just one or the other, this exercise combo is perfect for migraine fighting. With weight training, you can join a gym or buy free weights and other accessories for exercising in your home. To walk, of course, all you need are some good shoes and the great outdoors (or even a nearby mall).

Weight training tones muscles, improves muscular endurance, strengthens bones (thus fighting osteoporosis), lowers resting heart rate, and relieves stress. Walking is good for weight reduction, blood circulation, stress and pain relief, and overall health and endurance.

If you're just starting a walking program, aim for three times a week, and walk as far as you can comfortably handle. (Wiley Publishing's *Fitness Walking For Dummies,* by Liz Neporent, can help you get started.) If you can only walk a couple of blocks at first, that's okay. Pat yourself on the back for trying, and keep working to improve your stamina. You can gradually work up to longer distances over a period of months.

For tips on weight training, refer to *Weight Training For Dummies,* by Liz Neporent and Suzanne Schlosberg (Wiley Publishing), or get someone who's a knowledgeable bodybuilder or fitness professional to show you proper form and execution. Free weights and weight-training machines have to be used correctly in order to achieve gains. (Many people in the gym don't use weights or machines the right way. Then they can't figure out why they never make any progress!)

Fred Astaire your way to being headache-free

One 54-year-old headache sufferer took up ballroom dancing as a pain-relief complement to his prescription migraine pills and wound up competing in top hat and tails. "For me, it was a way to unwind from my high-stress job and try something radically different from anything I'd ever done before. The aerobic exercise worked wonders for me physically, and meeting new people was refreshing for me mentally."

His headaches decreased in frequency, and, as a fringe benefit, he found a wife on the ballroom circuit!

Shoot for doing a 45-minute weight-training session three times a week. If you combine a weight-training program with walking three to four times a week, you'll have a good migraine-combating exercise regimen. (Put workouts on your calendar or hand-held computer, just like you would any other important appointment. Make your health a top priority!)

You'll notice amazing improvements in muscle tone, self-empowerment, and confidence after only a few months of weight training. The gains may also motivate you to walk regularly for the aerobic benefits. The two exercises can be added to your regimen seamlessly.

Yo, can you say yoga?

Some movie stars swear by yoga. Moms-to-be take special pregnancy yoga classes. Older folks maintain their flexibility with the help of yoga poses.

And, indeed, some headache sufferers find that yoga works well for migraine relief and prevention. This form of exercise may serve as a worthy complement to other therapies you use for pain relief.

Yoga is believed to relieve stress, promote the release of *endorphins* (mood-boosting chemicals), and have a positive effect on the nervous system and digestion.

If you want to explore yoga, take a class at your local YMCA or a health club — or buy a how-to book, video, or DVD and just follow the example of the instructor. You can look for an instructor at The Yoga Site on the Internet at www.yogasite.com, which has a yoga teacher directory with listings for nearly every state in the United States as well as for countries ranging from Thailand to Iceland.

Yoga slows your heart rate and breathing as you do movements that stretch all of your muscles. Many believe that yoga enhances circulation and oxygenation throughout your body.

Trying Pilates, dancing, swimming, and skating

In your sampling of exercise options, you may want to try something you've never done before, such as some form of exercise that's ultra-trendy and sounds kind of fascinating. Ever consider dance classes? Swimming? In-line skating? Pilates?

Today's health clubs and gyms offer cool classes that go far beyond the aerobics-to-music that the early 80s ushered in. Now you can try kick-boxing, water aerobics moves, and cardio workouts that range from a traditional high-low aerobics combo to *step & sculpt* (a workout class that incorporates both stepping up on a bench and lifting free weights).

You can find classes, for all ages and levels of ability, for just about every type of exercise. If you're 60 and you're thinking of trying jazz dance, you won't have to worry about getting thrown into a class for teens. By the same token, you can find swimming groups for kids, young moms with babies, and seniors with arthritis. And just think, those nifty in-line skating kneepads can help you hide those unsightly knees that gravity has had its way with!

Sampling various types of dance can tell you what works for you. You may like ballroom, tap, jazz, or all three, but your headache-proclivity may not. Water exercise may appeal to you, but perhaps the chlorine acts as a migraine trigger. (Chlorinated chemical compounds have been linked to headaches.) Even something as harmless as the vibrations of in-line skates may aggravate your headaches, as your body is a delicately calibrated instrument.

One non-jolting form of movement that may suit you as a migraine sufferer is Pilates (pronounced "puh-LAH-teez"). Formerly used by professional dancers exclusively, Pilates is now a popular form of movement practiced in health clubs and dance studios all over the country. A few precise movements are performed in a certain order to strengthen and firm the body. You strengthen muscles between your hips and sternum as you improve your health without injuring yourself. By emphasizing muscle balance and strength, the instructor helps you increase your flexibility and develop a strong back and good posture. The reformer (Pilates equipment) accesses weak areas of your body so that you can work on improving alignment and balance.

Fine-tuning via physical therapy

You may discover that physical therapy can help relieve your headache pain, particularly if neck pain is a migraine trigger for you.

Physical therapists have quite a few options for putting headache pain at bay, but you must run the options past your physician before you participate in a physical therapy program (usually focused on the head/neck area). In fact, you need a prescription from a doctor to see a physical therapist.

You should keep your doctor abreast of every supplementary treatment or technique that you want to try, in order to have a well-coordinated and effective headache management plan.

The treatments that physical therapists offer are usually designed to reduce the severity and frequency of your headaches. Sometimes migraine sufferers visit physical therapists during a migraine attack, searching for a reprieve from the headache or from the neck pain that leads to migraines.

Some physical therapy options for migraines include

- **Multi-station electrical therapy:** The therapist stimulates trigger points — typically the earlobes and the loose skin between the index finger and thumb — with a *neuro probe* (an electronic muscle/neuromuscular stimulator) until they become somewhat painful. The therapist touches these points in an effort to break the cycle of pain.

- **Transcutaneous electrical nerve stimulation (TENS):** You can follow a do-it-yourself program by applying TENS with a battery-operated device, or you can have a physical therapist lead you through it. The device sends electrical impulses to electrodes that are placed where you have pain. Some people report reduced pain after about 15 minutes of stimulation.

- **Manual cervical (neck) traction:** The therapist supports your head as he applies a gentle, controlled force with his hands. The technique helps stretch and mobilize your spine.

- **Mechanical cervical traction:** If you find manual traction to be tolerable, but your headaches still persist, the therapist may apply mechanical traction, which takes the pressure up a notch or two. In mechanical cervical traction, a head halter with an attached weighted pulley system exerts force on your upper neck. You lie back into the equipment while you're lying on a table. Physical therapists find that this type of therapy often helps people who suffer from migraines that are aggravated by whiplash.

- **Vapo-coolant spray and stretch:** The therapist uses a fluori-methane spray (which acts as an anesthetic) on muscle groups, typically in the neck or upper back, where the pain is radiating to the head or neck. The spray blocks pain impulses (by making your skin cold) while the therapist stretches the muscles he thinks may be associated with your headaches.

- **Kinesiotaping:** Using a special physical therapy tape, the therapist tapes the whole length of the muscle group that is associated with your headaches in hopes of relieving any pressure that may be causing head pain. This therapy may be good for correcting the hunched posture that many people assume as a result of being in pain.

Here are some home remedies a physical therapist may recommend:

- **Moist heating pads:** You apply pads of moist heat to ease pain and improve mobility to your neck, head, or shoulder area.

- **Ice massage:** Here's a good migraine home remedy from physical therapist Charles Libby: Fill a paper cup three-quarters of the way full with water and freeze it. Take the frozen cup into the shower with you. Rip down the sides until half of the ice is exposed and only half of the cup remains. As you're pelted by the shower's warm water, rub your head with the ice. Add Ben-Gay to the water in the cup (before you freeze it) if you want to test the effect of this ointment along with the ice.

 ✔ **The hair pull:** Physical therapist Charles Libby grabs a few handfuls of the migraine sufferer's hair and then tightens his fist to place light traction on the head. He holds the patient's hair for 10 to 30 seconds. You can also try performing this remedy on yourself, or you can have a friend do it. (Make sure that it's a very good friend!)

Although some migraine sufferers report that physical therapy helps relieve their migraine pain, not enough studies have been done on the effectiveness of these treatments to establish their degree of helpfulness.

Massaging migraines away

Several types of massage can be helpful in relieving the pain of migraine headaches. But there aren't enough studies to show how effective — or ineffective — these therapies are. Typically, migraine sufferers who benefit from massage use it as one component of their pain-relief plan, along with medications, lifestyle changes, and so on.

You may want to give some of the following massage options a try:

 ✔ **Craniosacral therapy:** With this type of therapy, you lie back as a therapist gently massages your skull bones and your scalp. Your nerve endings get some touchy-feely attention, which soothes the nerves and lessens the pain waves they send.

 ✔ **Neuromuscular massage:** This therapy, which is also known as trigger-point therapy, is a muscle-relaxing treatment that applies moderate pressure to your body's *trigger points* (spots in a muscle that, when stimulated by pressure or touch, are painful). Some believe that it can reduce nerve compression and relieve pain in tense or overworked muscles.

 ✔ **Reflexology:** This therapy is based on the pressure and massage of points on the soles of the feet. The healing art of reflexology is often used to relieve stress and pain. For some headache sufferers, it's a godsend. It works on the idea that there are zones in the feet that correspond to all areas of the body. Therapists manipulate these zones, helping to benefit the corresponding areas throughout the rest of your body.

 ✔ **Deep-tissue massage therapy:** People get massages to get rid of pain and discomfort or to just give themselves a relaxing treat. A massage therapist uses pressure, movement, and stretching to render your body more pliable and comfortable. For headaches, a therapist will usually use therapeutic, deep-tissue techniques. Deep-tissue massages may serve to improve circulation and help reduce muscle tension. When performing a deep-tissue massage, a massage therapist focuses on specific areas of the body to relieve pain and release stress. Many believe that massage can reduce muscle pain and ease muscle tension and stiffness. *Deep* *tissue* refers to the use of deep finger pressure and slow strokes on areas of the body that are suffering from muscle tension or aches.

Because deep-tissue massage works well on tense shoulders and necks, it can sometimes provide relief from headache symptoms. (If you aren't sure whether your physical condition is amenable to massage, check with your doctor before having a massage. Massage isn't recommended if you have varicose veins, a recent fracture, sprain, or nerve injury, or if you've recently had chemotherapy or radiation.)

✔ **Acupressure:** For headache relief, acupressure techniques are used to apply gentle finger pressure to various points on your head. It is believed that this therapy can help headache sufferers by calming muscle tension and enhancing blood circulation. In a more ethereal sense, some think that acupressure promotes self-healing of the body by re-establishing energy balance. At any rate, this therapy is painless. So if you want to try it, check with your physician. (He'll probably give you a go-ahead.)

You can figure out how to perform a simple form of acupressure in minutes. Apply gentle and continuous fingertip pressure with two fingers for two to three minutes. Use one hand to work the top of your skull, and the other hand to apply pressure to the spot between your eyebrows. Of course, there are many other acupressure moves — you can get a book on the subject or have an acupressure practitioner take you through the steps.

✔ **Rolfing:** This therapy is one of many variations on the theme of massage. Its roots go back to the belief that most of us get all choked up with muscle contractions, which throws our bodies off balance. By applying deep pressure to your muscles, a Rolfing practitioner may be able to ease your headache pain by ratcheting down the tautness of your muscles. For some people, Rolfing reduces pain. For others, Rolfing is way too vigorous for their taste. We can put it this way: Rolfing is not for the person who's put off by aggressive body manipulation. (Basically, Rolfing is massage that is taken to a tougher intensity level. It's not a surefire headache remedy, by any means.)

The pressure of massage may cause some discomfort, but if you experience a great deal of pain, tell the therapist to stop. You may need to see your doctor for an evaluation.

Check with a local school of massage for the names of qualified therapists in your area. And when you're interviewing therapists, ask to see proof of membership in the American Massage Therapy Association (AMTA). Therapists with membership in this association have completed a training program approved by the Commission on Massage Training Accreditation/Approval, hold a state license that meets AMTA standards, and have passed an AMTA exam or the National Certification Examination for Therapeutic Massage and Bodywork. You can also find trained massage therapists on the AMTA Web site (www.amtamassage.org).

Avoiding Exercise that Induces Migraines

You love the butt-blaster aerobics class at your health club. Unfortunately, your head usually gets the biggest blast of all — a bolt of mega-pain that comes about after exertion. (Chapter 4 talks about exertion migraines.) The pain outweighs the gain. When you have to go home and nurse an awful headache, it certainly takes a lot of the fun out of your exercise efforts.

So what's a well-meaning fitness enthusiast to do? Two simple things: Know which types of exercise work for you, and know which ones work against you. In addition, you should keep in mind that warming up for at least 15 minutes may forestall exertion migraines.

If you can warm up sufficiently enough to get through major athletic events without migraines, good for you! But if you just keep having the same problem over and over, you have to understand that exercise extravaganzas just aren't for you.

Don't give up on exercise altogether. A regular exercise program is one of the best migraine deterrents of all.

Spinning, cycling, and aerobicizing your way to a migraine

Competitive cycling, Spinning (stationary cycling in a health club), and high-intensity aerobics classes are often headache-inducers for those who have a tendency to have migraines.

The names for aerobics classes have been ratcheted up to new levels of creativity, so you have to scrutinize the list of offerings to figure out which aerobics classes are the intense types. When checking out the descriptions of classes offered by health clubs, look for names such as "endurance workout," "step circuit," and "fat-burner." These classes are usually ones that are vigorous enough to have headache-spurring potential for migraine folks.

Some classes that you can probably handle without getting a headache are: yoga aerobics, pump (you lift free weights), stretch-and-move, hip-hop dance, and kick class (includes self-defense techniques).

You may be able to prevent migraines during these intense workouts if you participate in a long, slow warm-up before you begin. (See "Easing into exercise," earlier in this chapter, for warm-up suggestions.)

Toning down your running program

You want to run, but you get headaches every time you try. Here are some ideas for avoiding headaches when you run:

- ✔ **Warm up more fully.** You have to follow the same warm-up rule that other exercisers who get headaches must abide by — especially if you're often getting headaches from full-tilt running. Chances are, you already warm-up before you run. Now you're going to make your warm-ups even more extensive (perhaps a 15-minute walk prior to even the slightest trot).

- ✔ **Run shorter distances.** Cut down on your miles somewhat and see if it makes a difference.

- ✔ **Forget about running marathons and triathlons.** Look at what's really true for you — any form of running that involves over-the-top exertion may not be on your personal agenda, no matter how badly you want to run that marathon or be a champion triathlete.

Don't feel as though you're barred from running altogether. Just scale back your program, and be realistic about your boundaries. If you can have fewer, less-intense migraines, it will definitely be worth it.

Chapter 13

Eyeballing Environmental Enemies

*M*ore than you know. More than you'll ever know, you can be victimized by environmental creeps that instigate migraines. So one of your first missions is nailing your own personal triggers in your home, yard, and workplace. You may be exposed to such things as mold and dust mites — who knows what can be giving your brain's neurotransmitters and blood vessels a rough time? But, like other triggers in your repertoire, most of these can be handled. You can try simple remedies, such as using chemical-and-fragrance-free products in your home and changing air filters frequently — or you can go hog-wild and replace carpeting with ceramic flooring that's easier to clean and less of a haven for mold and dust mites.

Focus on environmental fixer-upper time. Find your culprits and send them packing! You can come up with endless creative ideas for environmental improvements that help get rid of migraine triggers. When making upgrades, remember that even if you discover that they really don't make your migraines less severe or less frequent, there's no downside to a cleaner environment.

Investigating Your Environment

When creating your overall migraine management plan, check for environmental triggers in your home, lawn, and workplace.

Migraineurs can be bothered by allegens such as dust, mold, and pollen; by changes in the weather or temperature; by glaring or fluorescent lights; and by strong odors and high altitudes — and even computer screens.

People who have migraines have a set threshold that, if exceeded, will result in a migraine. Any kind of upset — sleep deprivation, weather change, exposure to an allergen — can move a migraineur toward her threshold.

The following signs may indicate that your body is rebelling against something in your environment:

- ✔ Asthma or breathing problems
- ✔ Headaches
- ✔ Puffy eyes
- ✔ Rashes
- ✔ Runny nose
- ✔ Throat clearing (from postnasal drainage)

If you believe that environmental triggers are involved in your headache evolution, take the time to journal the places where you spend a lot of time, and see what trends you can spot.

Step one in environmental troubleshooting is pinpointing your personal triggers. You can discover your triggers rather efficiently by noting such information as when you experienced the migraine, where you were shortly before the migraine hit, and what you were exposed to in a particular room, building, or outdoor space.

You can use the headache journal in Chapter 3 when you're ready to journal environmental (and other) clues to migraines.

Kicking Troublemakers Out of Your Home

To start ridding your home of migraine gremlins, give your indoor environment a thorough critique, or hire someone to do this for you. An environmental inspector can evaluate your home and give you a list of recommendations for ways to eliminate toxins and improve the environment.

Take steps to eliminate as many allergens as possible — and, if needed, take an allergy medication to cut down on allergy symptoms, which can include headaches. Purify your drinking water, set up a schedule for frequent air-filter changes, and do some spring cleaning in your home.

The following list covers the most common indoor pollutants and tells you how to eliminate them or mitigate their effects.

- ✔ **Dust mites:** These microscopic-sized spiders live in pillows, mattresses, blankets, and other bedding. They're virtually invisible to the naked eye, and they feed on the dead skin scales of humans. Allergy symptoms are caused by the waste and body fragments of the mites, not the mites themselves.

To ward off dust mites in your home, be a cleaning wizard. Dust, mop, and vacuum often. Change the filters on your air-conditioning units often. Install air filtration devices to purify the air. Keep the humidity level low and the room temperature moderate, because mites thrive in warm, humid environments. (They can't survive at a humidity level that is less than 50 percent.) Change sheets, blankets, and bedspreads once a week, and wash them in hot water. You can also use zip-up covers on pillows and mattresses — this will hamper the mites' growth in bed dust.

Dry-steam vapor cleaning can deep-clean and sanitize your home without the use of chemicals. It removes dirt and kills dust mites, bacteria, and mildew.

✔ **Mold:** Keeping rooms on the dry side is a good mold preventive. Vent the clothes dryer to the outside of your house. Get rid of old books and mementos that can harbor mold. And stave off bathroom mildew with frequent and thorough cleanings.

✔ **Tobacco smoke:** Make your home a smoke-free environment, and ask all smokers to do their puffing outside. Smoking can really contaminate indoor air with formaldehyde, carbon monoxide, and other fumes. Smoke can also cause nasal congestion, headaches, bronchitis, and other health problems.

✔ **Carbon monoxide:** This colorless, odorless gas can come from tobacco, poorly ventilated fireplaces, wood stoves, gas appliances, burning charcoal, unvented kerosene heaters, or car engines running in your garage. It's poisonous, and it can cause symptoms such as fatigue, sleepiness, confusion, shortness of breath, headaches, heart and brain damage, and even death.

To control sources of carbon monoxide, make sure that any combustion process is well-ventilated. And ensure that each combustion device is as efficient as possible (see the manufacturer's instructions for how to accomplish this). You can monitor the levels of carbon dioxide in your home with a carbon monoxide detection device that plugs into a wall outlet. This device can be found at any home supply store.

If you want to go to extreme measures, replace all of your home's carpeting with ceramic flooring that won't harbor mold and dust mites. Wear cotton clothing, and swear off using chemical-filled products for bathing, grooming, or house-cleaning.

Checking Your Surroundings

Just by virtue of being a migraine sufferer, you're probably ultrasensitive to your surroundings. Lighting, smells, and even atmospheric pressure can affect you dramatically. Some of these things you can change. And some you have to live with. For example, barometric changes, high humidity, and heat can wreak havoc by touching off a headache spiral. But you can't control the weather. The only thing you can do is try to soften your exposure to the elements that upset your system.

In some people, environmental elements can trigger migraines, with symptoms of severe throbbing, nausea, light sensitivity, and other sensory disturbances.

Boring into buildings

If you keep an environmental journal, you may discover that the allergen that's kicking off your headaches is outside your home. Allergens outside the home often fall into the not-much-you-can-do-about-it realm. An environmental ogre in your workplace is especially daunting, because it's a trigger that you can't really escape — not unless you change jobs, anyway, and that's a pretty drastic solution.

The term *sick building syndrome* refers to a workplace that causes illness via agents in the air, with headaches often being one of the symptoms experienced (as well as nausea and dizziness). Depending on the cause, the symptoms can be treated, or you can avoid the physical factor causing the headache, if possible. You may want to ask to be relocated to another work site, or you may consider looking for another job if the company isn't willing to perform environmental troubleshooting.

If your company is amenable to the idea, you can suggest that they hire a consultant to come in and evaluate the building's environment. If your company declines, you may try offering to foot the bill (especially if you're the only one who's having headaches associated with the workplace). The inspector can provide ideas for improvements.

Caring about carpet chemicals

Indoor chemicals, such as gases from new carpeting in an office, can cause awful migraines. The carpet industry recommends ensuring good air quality via ventilating, choosing a low-emitting product, and cleaning.

Admittedly, some people report allergy-like symptoms after new carpet is installed. Typically, the emission level of new carpet drops within 24 hours of installation, and fresh-air ventilation can cause that level to dissipate within a few days.

To find out if a carpet, cushion, or floor-covering adhesive has been tested for emissions, look for a label showing that the product has undergone Carpet and Rug Institute Indoor Air Quality Testing. This label shows that the product meets stringent indoor air quality requirements for very low volatile organic compound emissions.

Visiting the Big Kahuna of environmental health

You receive a barrage of environmental input daily, and as long as the load is bearable, your body manages it efficiently. If the load becomes too much to handle, you may develop problematic symptoms, such as migraine headaches.

So maybe you're wondering how to get a once-and-for-all diagnosis of all your environmental baddies. The Environmental Health Center-Dallas (EHC-D) in Dallas, Texas, a facility that specializes in environmental medicine and works to solve difficult clinical problems, is one place that caters to people with this need (as well as others). The staff includes physicians, researchers, nutritionists, counselors, and other specialists. When patients visit EHC-D, their exposure to environmental triggers is limited. EHC-D boasts porcelain walls, Spartan décor, large air filters, and computers with screens that filter out electric fields. Patients are told not to wear perfumes. They must wear cotton clothing (no synthetic fabric) that has not been washed or cleaned in chemical products. Smoking isn't allowed, and, of course, the EHC-D is pesticide-free. Water is filtered to remove contaminants. Lighting is full-spectrum — no fluorescents. Flooring is hard surface only. (Carpet is notorious for harboring dust and mold.)

The staff of the EHC-D can test you for allergies to animal dander, molds, pollens, dust, food, and chemicals. They also perform electromagnetic sensitivity testing. After testing, you may receive treatment, which comes in several forms: immunotherapy with preservative-free antigens, autogenous vaccines, nutrition plans, nutrient therapy, energy balancing, psychological support services, and a chemical depuration program (combines dry heat, exercise, massage, vitamin replacement, and monitoring of toxin levels).

The doctors at the EHC-D search for the underlying environmental cause of illness. To find the underlying cause, they study the reactions of patients during their stay in the clinic. The stay usually lasts for about four to six weeks, a time frame that provides a window of opportunity free from home exposures. Upon leaving, the patient will know what lifestyle modifications should be made and what allergens need to be avoided. Some people may choose to model a "clean" room at home after EHC-D standards.

EHC-D also performs evaluations of homes and commercial buildings. They sell mold-testing kits for homes and offices. (For more information on EHC-D, call 214-361-9515 or 800-428-2343. You can also check your state environmental agencies for information on similar facilities that may be closer to where you live.)

While some allergists may tell you to get rid of carpeting if you have allergy headaches, it's not the carpet that causes you problems — dust, pollen, and mold spores can easily hide in your carpet. Using high-efficiency microfiltration vacuum bags (if you're using a vacuum cleaner with bags) or a vacuum with a HEPA (High Efficiency Particulate Air) filter can help get rid of these carpet creeps.

In some situations, changing the environment is out of the question. For example, if you're taking night classes at a community college, and something in the room is tipping off a migraine cycle, the school administrators probably aren't going to let you do a sweep of the premises to clean it up and make it less aggravating for you.

With this type of situation, your options are

- Living with the problem and taking an allergy medication
- Using a migraine pain relief medication when a migraine occurs
- Dropping the class so that you're no longer exposed to the offending allergen

Pulling up roots in your own backyard

Every time your husband barbecues on the grill, you end up with a migraine. The cause-effect process seems undeniable. So you must root around for the exact problem, and then do what you can to get rid of the trigger.

Consider the usual backyard migraine suspects: pollen, fumes from fresh paint, burning wood or charcoal, gasoline fumes from a car or lawnmower; fresh grass clippings, compost or leaf piles, and pet dander.

Pesticides and cleaning products can also add emissions to your environment. If you use such products, you should mop, sweep, or vacuum thoroughly afterward to reduce any residue left behind, making headache development less likely. Your lawn service may successfully kill the weeds in your lawn (and the fish in your local water) but grow a migraine in your head.

On safari for environmental big game

A woman we know suffered from migraines for 20 years. "I'd taken a million over-the-counter headache remedies, none of which helped much, and I was buying super-sized bottles of aspirin because I took about ten a day sometimes. Finally, I saw a TV newsmagazine show that recommended looking in your home for headache triggers."

She did just that, and she soon found that cleaning up her environment was just what she needed. She remembered that her internist had once mentioned the idea in passing, but she thought he was kidding.

"I decided not to expose my sensitive system to pollutants, so my mission was purifying my environment as much as I could. To eliminate dust in the air, I now change my air-conditioning filter once every two weeks, and I sleep on cotton sheets that I wash often in hot water. I got rid of products that were scented, and even changed to detergent and soaps free of perfumes. These things made a big difference — I rarely get a headache anymore except when I'm in some environment where I can't avoid chemical pollutants in the air, such as a friend's home."

Clean up your lawn areas so that you can feel comfortable sitting or playing outside. Zap the toxins and create a healthier outdoor environment for yourself (and your headache proclivity) and other family members, as well.

If you're just not sure what the problem is — but a headache always develops after you've been in your backyard (and it doesn't seem to be caused by glaring sunlight) — hire an environmental specialist to come in and inspect your lawn for problems and offer insight on the possible causes. (See the "Visiting the Big Kahuna of environmental health" sidebar in this chapter.)

Preparing a Personal Oasis

Maybe it's time to get your yin and yang in balance. Disharmony of your environment can be relieved somewhat by creating your own oasis, removed from the outside forces that lead to physical and emotional imbalance.

You can bet that Elvis had a place where he could go to unwind from his migraine pain. And while you may not need something on a grand scale, you can still benefit from setting up a home spa where you can spend some time being indulged and comforted by soothing smells, sights, and sounds.

You may even want to sample aromatherapy — and let your nostrils absorb some special scents that are renowned for their soothing properties. (See "Smelling your way to success with aromatherapy," later in this chapter.)

Springing for a home spa

What will help you relax when you feel like you're getting a headache? Think beautiful images. Fresh fruit on a tray. Pampering treatments. Home spa treatments are especially cool, because you can do them in your own home.

To create a home spa, look inward and discover the kinds of things that soothe you. "I hate the idea of all those candles around the bathtub, because I'm afraid something will catch fire," says one female migraine sufferer. Clearly, her spa setup should be candle-free. In other words, one woman's dreamy, posh bath is another woman's anxiety-producing water torture.

You can set up a total spa zone that's migraine-trigger-free. You may want your spa to come complete with all the fringe benefits — exercise equipment, sauna, whirlpool bath, and shower. Or your zone may be as simple as your bath space. Spa elements can be used to provide you with a getaway from daily stressors — it can be an occasional thing or something that you turn to regularly. Try to zero in on the types of spa phernalia that work for you, settle you down, and provide relaxation. You can use your spa as a migraine preventive or as a pain reliever when you have a headache.

Be sure to use chemical-free shampoos, conditioners, and bath products in your trigger-free zone. (You can buy these products in health food stores and specialty shops.)

A few ideas for soothing or pampering are

- **Setting the scene:** Put on some good music and place scented candles or fragrances around your spa space. Put drops of lavender essential oil in your bath. Set a tray of fresh fruit and a tall glass of water on the side of the bathtub.

- **Sloughing off:** Remove dead skin cells and regenerate your skin with a body *loofah* (a semi-abrasive body scrubber made from a sponge-like plant). Do a face steam-cleaning (apply a clean washcloth wet with warm water to your face four or five times, leaving it in place for several minutes), and use a masque made from equal parts raw oatmeal, honey, water, and olive oil. Then, after you wash it off, you can apply a mild moisturizer if your skin still feels dry.

- **Creaming those calluses:** For rough, callused heels, soak in your tub for 15 minutes and then get out and give them a vigorous sloughing treatment. Use a pumice and cream for foot exfoliation (both are available in drugstores and grocery stores). After you exfoliate, apply a rich moisture cream, put on socks, and luxuriate for an hour or so.

Just because a women's magazine tells you that a home spa should have certain elements doesn't mean you have to follow its suggestions to the letter. Do what works for you. Your migraine; your home spa.

Aromatherapy to go

If scents soothe your head, you can buy a locket that amounts to takeout aromatherapy. Feng shui consultant Judith Wendell offers AromaLockets, which are designed to diffuse three essential oils onto your skin via body warmth, over the Internet.

Another option for the road is an aromatic inhaler that is the size of a fountain pen and is filled with essential oils. You can choose from Wall Street Whiffer (red/peppermint), Rescue (green/eucalyptus), Unwind (brown/lavender), and HeartMender (blue/geranium rose). To order these aromatherapy products, visit the Sacred Currents Web site at www.sacred currents.com.

Smelling your way to success with aromatherapy

Aromatherapy is the use of plant oils — called *essential oils* — to soothe and enhance well-being. It's a fun treatment that's benign for most people when using most oils. (The exception would be someone who's allergic to a particular oil or fragrance.) Options in aromatherapy include potions, candles, shampoos, potpourri, and devices that hold essential oils.

Many healthcare providers remain unconvinced that aromatherapy is truly beneficial to your health, but the pleasing scents can relax you, and perhaps, reduce your anxiety (and thus, stave off headaches). Some people use aromatherapy for insomnia.

The essential oils lavender, peppermint, and chamomile are often touted as headache-soothers.

When you first use an essential oil, use only one drop on a tissue to make sure that you don't have an allergy or a bad reaction to it.

If you have skin allergies or asthma, or if you're pregnant, don't try aromatherapy until you clear the idea with your doctor.

You may want to have a certified aromatherapist treat you initially to demonstrate the proper technique and amounts. After the first treatment, you can do it yourself. To relax and ward off a headache cycle, try the following:

- **Compresses:** Hot and cold aromatherapy compresses are popular for relieving headaches. Put six to seven drops of essential oil in a cup of water and soak a washcloth in the solution. When the cloth is done soaking, place it on your aching head.

- **Steam inhalation:** Pour two cups of boiling water into a bowl and add six or seven drops of essential oil. Put a towel over your head to funnel the steam toward your nose. With your face about a foot away from the water, breathe deeply once, stop, and then inhale again. Do this exercise a few times.

- **Diffusion:** Spray an essential-oil/water solution into the air. You can buy spray units at gift and fragrance shops, or you can make your own by adding six to seven drops of essential oil to a cup of distilled water and pouring the solution into a spray bottle. (Remember to shake the bottle to distribute the oil before spraying).

- ✔ **Massage:** Some people like to use essential oils as part of a massage, rubbing them into the skin. You can buy massage oils at drugstores and some grocery stores.

- ✔ **Bath or Jacuzzi:** Add five to seven drops of essential oil to 1 ounce of carrier oil (a base), and then add the solution to your bath or Jacuzzi water.

Read the safety data for the essential oils you choose — there are safety precautions for each oil. Also, don't use essential oils for cooking! These oils aren't meant to be consumed internally. Some of them are poisonous.

Don't go overboard with scent sniffing. Too much of this good thing and you may get a headache!

Chapter 14

Looking at the Link between Migraines and Sleep

In This Chapter

▶ Looking for dysfunctional sleep patterns

▶ Knowing what you can change to avoid a migraine spiral

▶ Sampling remedies for sleep problems

Sleep can be a good remedy for migraines, but it can also be a migraineur's enemy. In many ways, slumber remains somewhat of a mystery, but at least one fact is clear: For those who have a headache tendency, having routine times for going to bed and getting up can help prevent headaches. Too much sleep, or too little, may lead to a migraine. Any type of off-kilter sleep (insomnia, sleep apnea, and so on) can spin off into a migraine.

Clearly, dysfunctional sleeping looms as a pivotal lifestyle factor that you can change to get your body back into a positive groove and help avoid migraines. When you reach the point where your sleep habits become reliable, you can cross sleep off your list of migraine-causing culprits.

Waking Up to Your Sleep Patterns

Although the exact amount of sleep a human being truly needs is basically an unknown, clearly some people can function perfectly well all day long after sleeping only 4 or 5 hours, while others grind to a slow meltdown on anything less than 10 hours. A baby may sleep 14 to 16 hours a day, while a senior (someone 65 or older) may average 5 or 6 hours a night. Apparently the older you get, the less sleep you need.

If you feel very sleepy during the day, you're probably not getting enough sleep at night, or your sleep isn't restful. You need quality sleep, and you need a sufficient amount.

Sleepless from Seattle to Sarasota

Consider the following findings from the 2002 Sleep in America Poll commissioned by the National Sleep Foundation (www.sleep foundation.org). This sleep-habit information (and many other factoids) was compiled from phone interviews of 1,010 adults:

✔ 27 percent characterized their quality of sleep as fair or poor.

✔ 58 percent reported having at least one of four symptoms of insomnia — waking up feeling fatigued, waking a lot during the night, waking too early and being unable to get back to sleep, or having difficulty falling asleep — at least a few nights a week. And 35 percent said that they had at least one of the four symptoms every night or almost every night during the previous year.

✔ 74 percent experienced at least one symptom of a sleep disorder a few nights or more a week. Symptoms of sleep disorders include the insomnia symptoms (see the previous bullet point), snoring, having pauses in breathing, and feeling an urge to move the legs when at rest (when you're lying down or sitting still).

✔ 15 percent of the respondents used a prescription sleep medication or an over-the-counter (OTC) sleep aid in the past year.

✔ 37 percent reported being so sleepy during the day that it interfered with daily activities a few days or more a month.

Many lifestyle factors can throw off sleep habits: You have the graveyard shift at work; a vacation turns your regular snooze routines topsy-turvy; a trip leaves you with jet lag; you sleep late on weekends to try to catch up on sleep you missed during the week; studying for finals keeps you up late.

One prevailing belief among sleep researchers is that the ups and downs of serotonin and its fellow brain transmitters during sleep may be what activate the road that leads to head pain. (Some migraine medications are used to regulate serotonin levels — see Chapter 8 for more info about these medications.)

Not surprisingly, erratic sleep habits are problematic for many migraineurs — chiefly because sleep problems are commonplace. Millions of Americans have trouble sleeping (see the "Sleepless from Seattle to Sarasota" sidebar for statistics), and lots of them are people who have to worry about headache triggers.

If you're migraine-prone, make establishing regular sleep patterns a prime focus of your headache management program. Establishing regular sleep patterns may be as simple as having more structure than in the past: You go to bed at the same time every night; you get up at the same time every morning; and you get the same amount of sleep regularly.

But harnessing sleep patterns may be more complicated if a sleeping disorder is instigating headaches. If you think that may be your problem, enlist a physician's help in evaluating and treating your sleep dysfunction.

Charting your sleep patterns

You already know whether your sleep tallies are all over the map. One night you get seven hours of sleep, the next night you catnap for two hours, and on Saturday you sleep ten hours. Your innocent little brain chemicals can't handle the craziness, so they report their distress by stirring up a migraine headache — they're crying out for orderly sleep habits!

Oversleeping is one of the top migraine triggers. That's why the bonus sleep hours that come with sleeping late on the weekend may kick off a headache. The other factor is that late-weekend-sleepers drink their first cup of coffee later than usual, allowing time for caffeine withdrawal to set the migraine roller coaster in motion. For some folks, daytime naps seem to initiate headaches; others find that napping actually helps zap headache pain.

To get to the bottom of poor sleep habits as migraine triggers, start a sleep diary and chart your sleep patterns for several weeks to see what you can discover. When you find your specific triggers, you can go to work on tweaking your sleep cycles.

When you wake up each morning, list the following things in your sleep diary (and keep track of them for about a week):

- What time you went to bed
- How long it took you to fall asleep
- How long you slept
- How you felt when you woke up (refreshed, tired, sleepy)
- How many naps you took during the previous day (and how long they were)
- Whether you woke up with a headache

By charting your sleep patterns, you can find out very quickly whether you sleep too little, too much, too restlessly, or too unevenly. You may even run across an easy fix — for example, if you find that napping during the day makes you wakeful and restless at night, you can eliminate napping.

Seeking help from sleep specialists

The specialists at sleep clinics are not migraine treatment specialists, but they can evaluate and treat sleeping disorders. The spin-off of their treatment may be a reduction in the frequency and severity of your migraines.

Sleep clinics have a staff of experts that usually includes a specialist in sleep-disorders medicine.

The clinics usually treat you as an outpatient. You undergo a physical exam, an interview, and, possibly, a screening test for psychiatric disorders. In some cases, the clinic may have you sleep in the laboratory for a night or two so that staff can track your sleep.

In a sleep study, your body's responses (brain waves, EKG, leg movements) are measured during night sleep. A doctor may also perform another study to measure the length of time it takes for you to fall asleep during day hours and your level of daytime sleepiness. Your healthcare provider uses this information to diagnose potential sleeping disorders.

When your body is hooked up to monitoring paraphernalia, sleep clinic personnel can chart your sleep periods, assess your medical information, and find the answers to the following questions:

✔ Are you actually getting a restless night's sleep?

✔ Are you sabotaging your own efforts to get to sleep? (Some activities, foods and beverages, and medications are counterproductive to restful sleep.)

✔ Do you have a sleep disorder?

✔ Can you benefit from treatment?

When selecting a sleep clinic, look for credentials from the American Sleep Disorders Association, which issues accreditation to clinics that meet its guidelines. To obtain a roster of accredited sleep disorder centers and clinics in the United States, call the American Sleep Disorders Association at 507-287-6006. (For more information on sleep disorders, visit the National Sleep Foundation Web site at www.sleepfoundation.org.)

Defining and Treating Sleep Disorders

To correct a sleep problem that leads to headaches, you need to first identify the nature of the problem. Just because you think that you have insomnia, it doesn't mean you know what's causing it or what you should do about it.

Certain sleep disorders can contribute to daytime sleepiness for the simple reason that you don't get enough sleep because you're tripped up by nighttime problems. To discover if your daytime sleepiness is the result of a sleeping disorder (and probably merits treatment), go through the following list to determine whether you frequently doze off or feel like you're going to fall asleep in the following situations:

✔ Watching television

✔ Listening to a speaker or sitting in church

- Reading
- Talking to someone
- Driving or riding in a car
- Sitting in a movie theater
- Eating at a restaurant
- Sitting at a computer
- Sitting at work

If you answered yes to several items in the list, your level of daytime sleepiness may be indicative of a sleeping disorder (especially if it's an ongoing problem), so you should seek evaluation. Chances are you may benefit from treatment.

Sleep disorders are more common in women, substance abusers, elderly folks, and people with mental and medical disorders.

If you have sleep troubles that you can't resolve, seek help from a doctor so that you can remove dysfunctional sleep from your migraine trigger list.

The following sections describe sleep disorders that can result in sleep loss and contribute to headaches.

Investigating insomnia

Although you may not be able to diagnose the more esoteric sleep disorders, such as sleep apnea or narcolepsy, you can easily identify insomnia. Check out the following list of symptoms:

- You have a hard time falling asleep even when you're tired.
- You often wake up in the middle of the night.
- You rarely feel rested when you wake up in the morning.
- You wake up much earlier in the morning than you need to for work or play.

If these symptoms sound familiar, you may have insomnia. In order to eliminate sleep troubles as a migraine trigger, you need to discover what's behind your insomnia.

Insomnia is the most common sleep problem. Many people experience a bout of insomnia at some point. Stress or a physical problem such as pain usually triggers the short-term version of insomnia. You may be caught up in the throes of worrying about a divorce, an upcoming exam, a business problem, money woes, health concerns, or illness or death of a family member, or you may just feel physically sick — you're having acid reflux from your stomach or your head hurts, for example.

Insomnia may last for only a few days or weeks; if it lasts for more than a few days, you need to investigate the underlying cause.

If you have *chronic* (long-lasting) insomnia, determining the underlying cause of your sleep problem before starting treatment is important. Chronic insomnia may result from a specific disruptive factor: Your house is by a freeway where the noise of passing cars never stops; your shifts at work frequently rotate from day to night; you have a medical condition that makes it hard to sleep; or the medication you take induces sleeplessness.

Some of the health problems that may cause insomnia are

- ✔ Anxiety disorders
- ✔ Arthritis
- ✔ Asthma
- ✔ Bipolar disorder
- ✔ Depression
- ✔ Gastroesophageal reflux disease
- ✔ Sinusitis
- ✔ Sleep apnea

Using drugs and alcohol can also contribute to an ongoing problem with insomnia. So can overusing sleeping pills or getting too much caffeine.

Insomnia treatments that may prove effective include getting out of bed when you can't sleep, using the bed for sleeping and sex only, avoiding daytime naps, relying on relaxation techniques, and taking sleep-inducing medication for short periods of time. If you don't discover an underlying cause for your chronic insomnia, you may want to try behavioral therapy. Studies suggest that behavioral therapy, in the long run, is more effective than taking sleep-aid medications.

Practicing somnambulism

Sleepwalking is more common in children than adults. Some people compare sleepwalking to bedwetting in that it's a problem most children outgrow.

When you sleepwalk, you take a nighttime stroll and don't remember it. You may get out of bed, move around the house, and even perform daytime acts such as eating, talking, dressing, or walking outside.

This temporary sleep malfunction happens when you're in a deep sleep stage. Because sleepwalking doesn't cause sleep deprivation, you probably won't need medical help for the condition.

People sometimes get hurt during these nocturnal wanderings. Treatment for children is usually protective in nature — keeping doors locked and having the child sleep in an environment where he can't hurt himself. Adults who sleepwalk may benefit from psychotherapy and medication.

Twitching your limbs

If you have *periodic limb movement disorder* (nocturnal myoclonus), you repeatedly move your arms and legs — especially your legs — while you're sleeping. These movements occur every 20 to 60 seconds and may make you wake up — or not. You may be completely unaware of the movements but feel sleepy during the day and wakeful at night.

Periodic limb movement disorder is typically diagnosed when a bedmate reports your activity. The disorder can be treated with exercise and medication.

Having lively legs

Restless legs syndrome is characterized by an uncomfortable or crawling sensation in your legs when you're trying to sleep. It's also described as an almost irresistible urge to move your legs. You may have this sensation when your legs are at rest and you're trying to go to sleep, but it can also occur with prolonged sitting.

You can usually relieve the sensation by getting up and moving around. Massaging your legs may help, too. Restless legs syndrome is often accompanied by periodic limb movement disorder. (See the previous section.) Both disorders are commonly seen in patients with migraine. Medications are available to treat restless legs syndrome.

Facing night fears

Night terrors disorder and nightmare disorder are two conditions that can be experienced on either a rare or frequent basis.

When you have a *nightmare disorder,* you wake up frightened by a scary dream. A nightmare (just like other dreams) is a phenomenon of REM (rapid eye movement) sleep. Nightmares may happen during high-stress times, or they may be experienced off and on, lifelong.

Typically, no treatment is required for nightmare disorder, because waking up from a nightmare usually is all that it takes to put you back on an even keel — you become reoriented quickly. However, if nightmares cause functional problems in your everyday life, a doctor will probably want to see if medication helps — for example, he may prescribe a tricyclic antidepressant drug that suppresses REM sleep.

Nightmares associated primarily with post-traumatic stress, a specific medical condition, or a side effect of a drug are different from run-of-the-mill nightmare disorder, because they're actually caused by a precipitating factor.

With *night terrors,* you not only wake up scared but you also yell and feel anxious and terror-stricken. Night terrors are most often seen in children. In rare cases, night terrors may be a sign of temporal lobe epilepsy; your doctor may want to do neurological tests to determine if you have this disorder.

Treatment for both nightmare disorder and night terror disorder can range from simple reassurance to medications.

Falling asleep fast and frequently: Narcolepsy

Narcolepsy causes sleep attacks, during which you fall asleep like a curtain falling. When you have these attacks, you may stay asleep for varying lengths of time (anywhere from a few seconds to 30 minutes). The attacks can happen anytime, whether you're walking down a path, talking to someone, or sitting in church.

Narcolepsy is sometimes accompanied by *cataplexy,* which is a sudden loss of muscle tone brought on by an emotional stimulus, such as laughter or surprise. With cataplexy, you may experience weakness in your legs or paralysis of muscles (causing a collapse), or your jaw may drop. If you experience muscle paralysis, you may be unable to speak or move.

Narcolepsy, which is usually considered a result of a central nervous system abnormality, can be managed with drug therapy. If you suspect that you have narcolepsy, it's very important to seek treatment. Without treatment, you put yourself and others in jeopardy (especially when driving).

Taking a break from breathing with sleep apnea

Loud snoring? Morning headaches? Extreme fatigue? Daytime sleepiness? All are signs of *sleep apnea,* a condition where your breathing stops for 10 seconds or longer during sleep. It often occurs many times throughout the night.

Snoring, a common symptom of sleep apnea, refers to the noisy breathing that results from the vibration of soft tissue at the back of the mouth. Snoring may be caused by drooping tissue, large tonsils and adenoids, or obstructed nasal airways. In children, loud snoring and obstructive sleep apnea are usually caused by enlarged tonsils or adenoids. Surgical removal of the tonsils or adenoids can solve these problems.

Sleep apnea can be life-threatening, resulting in problems that range from heart attacks to car accidents (from the daytime sleepiness). Seek treatment from a sleep specialist or an otolaryngologist (ear, nose, and throat doctor), who will examine your nose, throat, neck, and palate. He may also order a *polysomnography exam* (a sleep study).

Treatments for sleep apnea include weight loss, avoidance of sleeping on your back, an oral device during sleep, cervical support pillows, treatment for nasal obstruction, surgical removal of tonsils, laser surgery, and a mechanical breathing device called a CPAP (continuous positive airway pressure) machine. The *CPAP machine* is used to open the throat during sleep — a mask goes over the nose, and a pump keeps the airway open via air pressure.

Sampling specific sleep remedies

Sleep aids can reduce the time it takes for you to fall asleep and make it less likely that you'll wake during the night. On the other hand, sleep aids may make you feel drowsy the following day and cause problems with withdrawal when you stop taking them — insomnia all over again.

Making use of medications

Sleep medications are usually recommended for short-term use only (if at all).

For short-term insomnia, your doctor may prescribe a sleep medication such as Ambien or Sonata. Medications called benzodiazepines may also be prescribed for short-term use.

You may also want to try eating a bedtime snack that's high in the amino acid tryptophan — it will help make you drowsy. Milk and yogurt are both high in tryptophan.

People with depression often experience improved sleep after taking an antidepressant for a few weeks. However, antidepressants can also cause insomnia.

Make sure that you have your doctor review your current medications before you take anything to induce sleep. Sleeping pills can sometimes be a huge health hazard when combined with other drugs or medical conditions. If you're 60-plus, the risk is even greater, because your nervous system may be ultrasensitive and your body slow to process medicine.

Tuning in to melatonin

Some studies suggest that the dietary supplement *melatonin* — a synthetic version of a hormone your body produces naturally — can sometimes help people develop normal sleep patterns. How does it work? The melatonin in your body is produced in the pineal gland at the base of your brain. When the production of melatonin goes up, your alertness is reduced, and your temperature falls. Your natural melatonin levels are low during the day, but they increase at night. Bright light inhibits your pineal gland's melatonin secretion (so sleeping with a light on isn't a good idea).

You have more melatonin as a child than you do as an adult (and even less when you get old).

You can buy melatonin at grocery stores, health food stores, and drugstores. Unfortunately, the wild cattle call in the '90s that caused millions of Americans to line up for "miracle melatonin" did a great deal of harm. Touted as a cure for aging, a treatment for jet lag, and a perfect solution for insomnia, melatonin failed to live up to the hype. Many of the people who tried it were disappointed. So lots of Americans dismissed melatonin the minute they found out that the pills weren't really instant problem solvers.

If you decide that you want to use melatonin as a sleep aid, take it only under medical supervision, and don't take it at all if you're pregnant. Your doctor probably won't want you to take it for more than four weeks.

Makers of melatonin are not allowed to say that it cures or treats disease, but they can say something general — such as that it's a good sleep-inducer. Also, you should know that melatonin hasn't been tested extensively. Because it's not sold as a drug, manufacturers don't have to list its side effects on the label. Some users report side effects of depression and hallucinations.

Benefiting by Changing Your Behavior

A therapist can guide you in altering behaviors that contribute to poor sleep patterns. Improving your sleep patterns can help you get rid of a lifestyle factor that may be a migraine trigger.

Your goal is to get rid of nonproductive behaviors that lead to sleep problems, and substitute new behaviors that will, hopefully, allow you to eliminate the sleep problem that may be spurring your headaches.

You decondition yourself away from certain ways of thinking — using the bed as a place to work or watch TV, for example — and condition yourself to a new way of thinking (that your bed is only for sleeping and sexual activity).

When you work on mentally reframing your sleep situation, you may want to use the following methods:

- **Rethink the role of your bed.** Desensitize your fondness for using your bed as a recreation area. Look at your bed as a sleeping place (not a do-all, end-all activity spot).

- **Try stimulus control therapy.** The goal is to change your nonproductive sleep behaviors. Some recommendations for changing your sleep behaviors are: using the bed only for sleep and sex; getting out of bed when you can't fall asleep and doing a calming activity such as reading; and trying to wake up at the same time each morning, no matter how many hours you sleep. (Don't go to extremes, though; a little sleep deprivation will be beneficial with this treatment, but a total lack of sleep can impair your ability to drive a car, and so on.)

- **Use self-talk to banish your anxiety about sleep.** If you go to bed and immediately start worrying that you're going to have trouble sleeping, adopt the practice of using self-talk that is upbeat: "I will soon start feeling sleepy. I am going to fall asleep soon. I no longer will have trouble with sleep. Sleep is going to flow as easily as breathing." Also, if your mind wants to rehash problems during the night, have a line ready to push it away: "I can't do anything about that problem during the night, so I won't think about it right now."

- **Do progressive muscle relaxation.** Tense and then relax your major muscle groups by starting with the ones in your feet and moving up your body to your head. Some doctors recommend biofeedback to relieve muscle tension and stress (see Chapter 9).

- **Try role-playing.** You take yourself through the steps of going to bed, relaxing, and imagining yourself falling off to sleep and waking up rested in the morning. You practice going back to sleep after you get up during the night to go to the bathroom, or when you wake up and your mind starts buzzing. You manage your fears ("I won't get enough sleep to go to work!" "I'll never get back to sleep!") by replacing them with self-affirming outcomes: "It doesn't matter if I wake up during the night; I'll lull myself back to sleep in seconds."

- **Improve your sleep hygiene.** Avoid caffeine and late meals, and avoid or limit your alcohol consumption. Also, try to improve environmental problems, such as excessive noise and light, and uncomfortable room temperatures.

✔ **Stay positive.** Quit beating yourself up — don't ridicule yourself as a "goofy, lame, pitiful nonsleeper." Being unable to sleep isn't tragic or the end of the world. Think of it as "a problem in living." Be optimistic about improving the situation, and you'll be successful.

Fixing lifestyle habits that hamper your slumber

If you have sleep deficiencies or disorders, you need to be careful to exercise, eat a healthy diet, and keep from throwing your body any curves. In fact, you can make some simple lifestyle changes that may correct your sleep troubles with relative ease.

You need to know what not to do, so that you can avoid driving off into those gutters. The following are some common habits that can lead to herky-jerky sleep patterns:

✔ **Consuming foods or beverages that contain too much caffeine:** Don't drink or eat anything that contains caffeine within three hours of bedtime. Avoid alcoholic drinks and hot chocolate; both are rumored to be good for helping you sleep, but they can actually be migraine triggers. Chocolate can serve as a stimulant within a few hours of consuming it, and alcohol can cause you to be wakeful during the night.

✔ **Pigging-out late at night:** You can have a light snack before bedtime, but avoid eating a big meal after 7 p.m.

✔ **Using illegal drugs:** Illegal drugs such as cocaine or amphetamines can cause a wide-awake state (and other more serious problems). The answer is simple — stop using illegal drugs.

✔ **Taking medications that can affect sleep:** Ask for your doctor's help in looking over your medications to see if any of them have the side effect of acting as a stimulant or interfering with your sleep in some other way. Some common sleep-curbing offenders include: diet pills, diuretics, prescription or over-the-counter drugs containing caffeine, nasal decongestants, steroids, some antidepressants, and certain asthma and blood pressure medications.

✔ **Overusing sleep medications:** This is one of the most common causes of sleep problems. The notorious rebound problem that plagues migraine sufferers when they overuse pain medicines can be paralleled by overdoing sleep meds: You take so many sleeping pills that you eventually have to take more to receive any sleep-inducing benefits. After a while, you begin to establish a dependency on these medications.

✔ **Sleeping with a partner who snores:** You can grab your pillow and sleep in a different room or try to find a way to correct the snoring (that's another book!). If you sleep with a person who snores, a nudge in the ribs and a "please turn over" may nip the problem in the bud. The snorer, when repositioned, may stop snoring. However, if the person snores excessively or has episodes in which he briefly stops breathing, he needs to see a healthcare provider to be evaluated for sleep apnea. (See the "Taking a break from breathing with sleep apnea" section, earlier in this chapter, for symptoms of sleep apnea.)

✔ **Exercising right before bedtime:** If possible, schedule your exercise program for morning or afternoon. Avoid any kind of vigorous exercise just before sleep, because your body may get revved up and keep you from falling asleep. We don't recommend a sedentary lifestyle. Regular exercise definitely promotes sound nighttime sleep and steady sleep patterns. (See Chapter 12.)

✔ **Sleeping in an environment that's not conducive to relaxation:** This sleep antagonist has a simple solution: You just figure out what's bothering you and fix it. If the room is too quiet, get a ceiling fan — the nice hum will help you sleep. If your bed is too hard, too soft, or otherwise uncomfortable, buy a mattress pad or a new mattress. Replace your worn-out pillow. Play soft music to dull sounds coming from nearby houses or apartments. Keep the temperature at a comfy level.

You can also set up a dreamy bedroom. If it takes a lacy canopy to make you feel soothed and sleepy, put one over your bed. If you want to sleep in total darkness, use heavy drapes and shades on your windows. To get rid of irritating noises, buy a white-noise machine or do what you can to sound-proof your sleep setting.

✔ **Smoking tobacco:** People who smoke often suffer from disrupted sleep. Therefore, this is just one more reason you should stop smoking.

✔ **Experiencing arthritis pains:** Check with your doctor for ways to relieve any aches and pains that wake you up during the night. It may be as simple as taking an OTC medication such as Aleve.

Doing sleep things differently

If you want to avoid the migraine spiral that gets jumpstarted by your erratic sleeping, you have to improve your slumber situation by managing healthier sleep.

Here are things you can do to reset your body clock for success and avoid the migraine spiral:

✔ **Learn how to wind down.** Just like a child who won't go to sleep after a few minutes of rough-housing right before bedtime, you may have trouble shifting from high to low gear. Find a way to soothe yourself into a peaceful mode. Take a long, warm bath. Drink a glass of warm milk. Use a relaxation technique before you go to bed: Take yourself through muscle relaxation, starting with your toes and moving up to your head (see Chapter 9).

✔ **Get out of bed when you can't sleep.** When you can't sleep, get up and read or watch TV. If you lie in bed and think, "I need to get to sleep because I've got to go to work tomorrow," you can produce exactly what you don't want — a wide-awake state of worry and stress. Try not to think too much about your sleeplessness or turn your inability to fall asleep into a big deal. If you're not sleepy, you can't go to sleep, so why try? And if you can't fall asleep even though you're sleepy, vow not to fret about it. Just get up and do something, and then return to your bed when your eyelids are feeling heavy and you suspect that your body is ready to let you fall asleep.

✔ **Avoid the nap syndrome.** Sleep labs reveal that people who take day-time naps often have abnormal nighttime sleep patterns. So if you're experiencing poor sleep at night, don't give in to the impulse to take a catnap in the afternoon. (The exception to this rule is older folks, who probably need to nap.)

If you're having problems with insomnia, don't nap in an attempt to make up for lost sleep. Your body will be sure to soak up some extra deep sleep the following night to make up for what you lost.

✔ **Don't pop a pill.** Don't take any form of sleeping medication without consulting with your doctor. (If your doctor tells you it's okay to use sleeping pills, do so very seldom and use the smallest dose that's effective.) Sleep medications may even make it harder for you to sleep or give you a drugged feeling the next day. You can also become psychologically or physically dependent on some sleep drugs.

Don't drink alcohol when you use a sleep medication. It can add to the sedative effect of the drug. Instead, just let the sleep med do the trick for you.

✔ **Get enough sleep:** Get enough sleep to help you feel refreshed and ready to seize the day, but not so much that you feel groggy and lethargic.

Improving your child's unstructured slumber patterns may eliminate his sleep problems as a migraine trigger (see Chapter 20). Children with migraines show specific benefits from the correction of erratic sleep habits — they tend to have fewer and shorter experiences with migraines. Improvement in their headaches apparently stems from cutting down on end-of-day caffeine consumption, increasing nighttime sleep hours, and following consistent wakeups and bedtimes.

Part V

Staying Connected to the People in Your Life

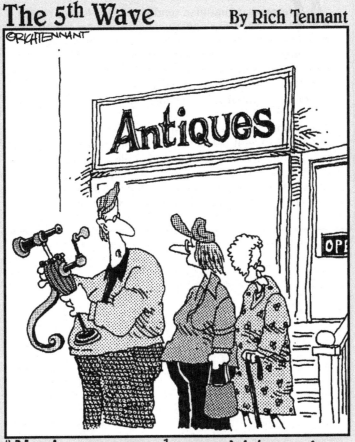

The 5th Wave   By Rich Tennant

Antiques

"Marsha, come over here and let me show you what my migraines feel like."

In this part . . .

Migraines sometimes send you to the locker room. Pain and other migraine symptoms can bump you out of the game temporarily, and the people around you — your mate, children, boss, co-workers, in-laws — may not know how to interpret your being out of commission. This part shows you how to cope with these folks and reduce your anxiety when you're dealing with chronic headaches.

A migraine can be an irritant for sure, but because you're not about to let it detract from the glorious experience of living, you need to find ways to handle migraine isolation at work, keep your family on the same page, and accept the attitudes of people who just don't understand migraines. This part helps you do just that.

Chapter 15

Living the Good Life Despite Migraines

So what's a migraineur supposed to do while she's waiting to get better? The enormity of the disability aspect of migraines is enough to take your breath away, not to mention mess with your mind. Plagued frequently with an aching head, you may feel dazed and confused, flummoxed and fragmented, conflicted and conflagrant. But, the truth is, you can live a normal life despite sometimes being hobbled by high-level pain.

You don't have to write off the fun part of life just because you suffer from migraines. Far from it. You only need to make a few adjustments to make sure that your nights of revelry aren't followed by days of blinding misery. You can discover how to deal effectively with the inevitable migraine blues. If you need to, figure out when it's best to become a migraine recluse — just go to bed and sleep off your pain. Figure out how to have fun despite the head-pain drawback. And hold on to your patience when migraine-free folks act like they think you're faking it.

Singing the Why-Me Migraine Blues

Migraines may make you feel sad and lethargic. Your appetite may be next-to-nothing, and you may have trouble sleeping. You may tell people close to you that you're depressed, because it's the only word you know that accurately describes the low mood of persistent head pain.

Switching focus to lose the blues

If you've had headaches for many years, you may be familiar with the migraine blues. But are you good at dealing with it?

A nurse we know found herself steeped in self-loathing every time she had to miss work with a migraine. She loved her job and hated the disability aspect of her headaches. "One day I decided I was going to fix my migraine grumpiness," she says with a laugh. "I knew I was driving my husband crazy, the way I grumbled all the time."

She sought the help of a psychotherapist, who asked her the hot-button question: "Do you really think you're worse off than most people?" "I felt so silly," recalled the nurse. "One of my friends has breast cancer, and another is going through the enormous stress of a lawsuit. Yet another is getting her third divorce." She admitted to the therapist that several of her friends had worse problems. "But knowing that really doesn't help," she said. "Getting outside yourself will help, though," the therapist said. "Look at some volunteer opportunities, and pick one. Then, make time for it. When you're feeling down about your migraine burden, go to the volunteer center and help some really unfortunate people."

She took her therapist's good advice and found that helping others did change her feelings about her own lot in life. "I still don't like having migraines, but I know how to shake the gloomy, blue feeling. Helping other people makes me focus less on myself. That makes all the difference in the world. I highly recommend trying this kind of thing."

Don't be afraid to give yourself permission to hate migraines. After all, you'll only be in major denial if you try to pretend that you aren't irritated by having horrible headaches now and then. In fact, dealing with depression (or the blues) is an almost inevitable spin-off of being a migraineur. Anyone with any chronic illness (which migraines are) is at risk for depression. Researchers believe that having migraines may make you more susceptible to developing depression. And the flip side is true, too: Having depression makes you more likely to have migraines.

Don't be surprised (or frightened) if your doctor prescribes Elavil — an antidepressant that is good at fighting depression and excellent for busting migraines. Antidepressants are not only used for fighting depression, they're also commonly used to treat people with migraines.

If you're having symptoms of clinical depression, you need to see a doctor immediately. These symptoms include

- ✔ Despondent mood
- ✔ Disinterest in normal activities
- ✔ Fatigue and low energy level

✔ Feelings of worthlessness or guilt

✔ Indecisiveness or inability to focus

✔ Insomnia or *hypersomnia* (sleep that lasts for long periods of time)

✔ Restlessness or a feeling of general slowness

✔ Significant weight loss or changes in appetite

✔ Suicide plans or attempts

✔ Thoughts of death

If you have five or more of these symptoms in a two-week period, to the extent that they interfere with your ability to function adequately and represent a change in your life that isn't the result of drug abuse, a medication, a medical condition, or a natural grieving process following the loss of a loved one, get evaluated immediately.

Feeling Free to Get Pain-Free

Don't be afraid to take aggressive moves when battling migraine pain. Some people, despite their migraine misery, don't feel entitled to pull out all the stops when trying to nix head pain, mainly because of the stigma attached to drug use. Plus, they may fear that taking a strong pain reliever will make them feel even worse (the "dull brain" haze). Many people use heavy-duty medications to fight headaches. If these drugs work for you, don't let the stigma of the drug's name or strength level hold you back.

You may find it daunting to take antidepressants (the ones used to fight migraines) or seriously strong painkillers, because you feel like you're giving in to the fact that you need a formidable drug to knock out your headache. Remember, though, that lots of people have to take strong medications to keep medical conditions at bay or reduce symptoms of chronic illnesses. It's nothing to be ashamed of — just real life.

When deciding to take a heavy-duty drug, you should consider

✔ How well the drug works for you

✔ How tolerable its side effects are for you

✔ How liberating the effect of being migraine-free will be, thanks to the drug

Don't feel bad about occasionally using heavy-duty medication if that's what it takes to get rid of some of your headaches. After all, that's what these drugs are for. Just make sure that you follow your doctor's instructions for using the drug, and don't increase your dosage or your frequency of taking it.

If you're lying in your bedroom writhing in headache pain, it's no time to be reticent about pain relievers.

It's a good idea to have your doctor on board when making all decisions concerning medications for headaches and any other treatments you may try, from herbal supplements to chiropractic treatments. You can feel safer and more secure with your physician monitoring your progress and answering your questions about side effects.

Deciding Whether to Go Out and About or Hunker Down at Home

One the most difficult tasks for a migraine sufferer is figuring out how to deal with everyday life when suffering from a splitting headache. You ask yourself, "When can I manage a headache with medication and still get out of the house to do a few things? And when should I just forget about trying to do anything and fall into bed for sandman therapy?"

Knowing when it's okay to leave the comforts of home is a key part of migraine management — it's not always an easy call. How can you tell if a course of action on a headache day is doable? The following list gives you some tips for gauging your prowess at taking care of business when dealing with a headache:

- ✔ **Assess your attitude for the day.** Don't take part in regular workplace or home activities unless you're pretty sure that you can stay on an even keel. (If you're going to be cranky with co-workers or your kids, you may be better off waiting until you shake the headache).

- ✔ **Determine exactly why you're trying to get out and about.** If you're truly miserable with pain, but you feel like you have to strive for super-parent or super-worker status, stay home. You probably won't be able to accomplish anything, anyway; if you do, the effort will be at your health's expense.

- ✔ **Evaluate the effects of your medication on your ability to function.** Don't indulge in work or family errands or duties if your migraine brain haze can jeopardize your or someone else's safety: You should drive only if you have a clear head when you're taking your migraine pain medication. (If in doubt, check with your doctor to get his opinion on the safety of driving when you're taking a certain medication.)

Basically, your own personal experience will teach you what's workable with your pain-severity level. You may find, over time, that taking a pain reliever and then going about your usual routine can have a pain-relieving effect. Or you may have the opposite experience — discovering that your pain gets worse with any kind of activity.

Sleeping off a migraine

You may find that taking pain medication and sleeping off a migraine is the perfect remedy for your migraine pain.

If sleep works wonders for your head pain, don't hesitate to get some extra sleep. The fact that you sometimes snooze away migraine pain doesn't make you lazy, reclusive, or any of the other adjectives that an outsider may come up with. For you, a timeout or a day off may simply be the smart answer.

Give yourself permission to do what you need to do. Take care of the business of getting rid of your headache. If freeing yourself from outside noise, light, and household confusion helps, it's definitely the right way to go. Snuggle up in a comfortable bed and let some good Z's bring you sweet release from your migraine.

Taking care of business with a monkey on your head

Thousands of migraineurs go to work with headaches. Thousands of stay-at-home moms continue car pools and grocery-store trips, even though they're suffering from headaches. Lots of people conduct board meetings, close deals, and give seminars while dealing with headaches.

Here are some coping strategies for days when you have not-quite-incapacitating headaches:

- ✔ Take an over-the-counter medication that takes the edge off your pain.
- ✔ Keep the reassuring self-talk coming. ("I can run this errand and then go home and go to bed.")
- ✔ Set parameters for yourself. ("I won't try to work on that major presentation today; I can get through the simple stuff, but it would be foolish to tackle anything that requires extreme focus.")

Joining in the Social Whirl

From the time you were first diagnosed with migraines, you probably wondered exactly what it would mean for your social life. Do migraines automatically send you to the world of social nerdiness? Not necessarily. Actually, you can decide what you want to do and be, and then set your sights on finding a way to do those things. Thousands of migraineurs do it all the time.

Sure, sometimes you may have to cancel things. Feeling a bit of chagrin is natural, but remember that many people bail for other reasons, such as a virus, menstrual cramps, a family emergency, or food poisoning — the list goes on and on. So it's really not all that bad if you have to cancel sometimes.

Dating and mating

You set up a date, the big evening arrives, and those nasty migraine triggers team up and throw you a curve that escalates into massive head pain. You know that there's no choice but to take your migraine medication and go to bed — after calling your date to say, "I can't go anywhere tonight."

If the person you're canceling on happens to wind up as your significant other, she'll have to live with your migraines long-term, so why not see how her affection holds up from the get-go?

Everyone has problems that they cope with long-term. So try to have a sense of humor about having to cancel a date when you're suffering from a migraine. Tell your date that you feel bad — you have a migraine — but you'd like a rain check. Make it clear that the headache isn't an excuse — it's a reality.

You're going to be bummed, sure, but you can show an upbeat attitude: "When I have one of these, I usually feel better the next day, so I hope we can reschedule. It doesn't take long for me to get sick of being a shut-in!"

Partying down despite a party-pooper migraine

You *can* party. Yes, you can. "With monkeys biting my head?" you ask. How is it possible to love the nightlife when you're shuddering in a fit of pain? Is it really within the realm of reality?

Yes, you can sparkle, crack jokes, yuck it up, and do Britney Spears dance moves — *if your headache is on the way out.* Essentially, the only thing you have to do is decide if you feel like you can party hearty and enjoy yourself. If not, don't push yourself, and don't go into denial; listen to your body talk.

If alcohol is a known headache trigger for you, avoid alcoholic beverages. Of course, you can expect a date (or mate or gal-pal) to urge you to "have just one," but stand your ground. You don't want to end up with a hammering head.

Get creative, and find a way to let your saucy party-self get out there when you do feel good. Make the most of your situation — don't be afraid to shake your bootie!

Turning thumbs down on fireside chats

One migraine sufferer in an online support-group chat room said something that non-migraine folks may find unbelievable. "When I go on ski trips, I always get headaches sitting by the cabin's fireplace."

This statement only goes to illustrate the quirkiness of migraines. Something as seemingly innocent, benign, and delightful as a fireside evening carries at least three possible migraine triggers: hot chocolate, hot toddy, and the smell and smoke of the wood fire.

The message is this: Find out what can bother your system, and honor your body's preferences. If you're just dying to try something that you're unfamiliar with, be sure to have your migraine medication ready to go. Don't get caught unprepared!

Finding recreation you can enjoy

Thrash around for fun opportunities! If you're a migraineur whose system is easily nudged into Painsville, be sure to seize chances that allow you to make the most of your uptime.

People with migraines usually develop a heightened appreciation for enjoying every single day because of their great awareness of the potential for many hours of downtime.

For every activity that you can't tolerate, there are literally thousands that you can tolerate. All you have to do is eliminate those few that you can't handle!

Intense aerobic activities are often troublesome for migraineurs, so you may not be able to soar as a snow skier, a triathlete, or a mountain climber. But you probably can be a dancer, a swimmer, a skater, a fast walker, a hiker, a yoga enthusiast, a knitter, or a gardener.

Here are some ways to weigh the headache potential for a recreational activity:

- ✔ **Consider the weather and setting:** Will the activity feature changes in altitude and weather, both of which are often migraine triggers? One study suggests that half of all migraines have weather changes as an ingredient in their inception.

- ✔ **Review the specific environment of the activity:** Will there be bright lights, loud noises, and strong fumes? A concert, for example, may merit your no-no list (unless you think ahead and make sure that you're not sitting by the speakers).

You can enjoy more recreational activities by working around things that may affect your migraines. For example, say that you're going to a birthday party in a Mexican restaurant, and avocados are on your migraine trigger list. You can simply take the alternative route of stuffing your soft corn tortillas with chicken, refried beans, and rice, and steer clear of guacamole, which is made with avocados.

Keeping It Real When Migraine-Free People Think You're Faking It

Occasionally, someone you encounter may doubt the reality or severity of your headaches. It happens. You have to live with it. You can't go through decades of migraine living and escape headache skeptics altogether.

Ignore any and all snide comments about your headaches. Exploding every time someone makes a rude remark about your migraine problem is unproductive, and it only makes matters worse.

Case in point: You're visiting in-laws, and everyone is sitting down for Christmas Eve dinner. Wineglasses are accenting place settings all around. You watch your sister-in-law snatch up your wineglass and make the curt comment, "Well, of course you won't need this, because you always have a headache." *Ouch.* You can't help but feel injured by her words — and the insinuation that you're a no-good wimp who's fabricating the whole migraine thing.

So what's the proper response? Naturally, you feel outraged — how can anyone think that you'd fabricate your migraine suffering? It's important to keep your response simple: "No, I won't be having any wine." Smile and remember that you have nothing to gain from a skirmish or confrontation, especially not with relatives. Remind yourself that people who don't have migraines don't understand them!

Most people know very little about migraines unless they, too, are sufferers. You may also find that most people don't want to know anything about migraines. If you're ever in doubt about the wisdom of filling people in on migraines, think about your dear old aunt who responds to "how are you?" with a full-blown account of her latest, greatest bowel movements. *Don't go there.* The truth is, some subjects just aren't worth pursuing with disinterested parties.

A marketing executive who has suffered from migraines for 30 years tells how her husband always jumped in and smoothed things over for her when she had to exit a party because of a migraine. "He would say something sweet like 'I can always tell when my beautiful wife is getting a migraine, because her hair goes flat.'" After that, people kindly tut-tutted her suffering, and no one ever offered a skeptical word or look.

Chapter 16

Managing Migraines at Work

*Y*our boss had you at hello. That is: "*Hello!* Do you expect me to believe you have *another* migraine?"

The enormity of the workplace migraine issue simply can't be overestimated — something you're all too familiar with if you've lived with headaches for a number of years. You may wish that you could wear a MedicAlert bracelet or a get a big "M" tattoo — anything that would warn people in advance that you have real headaches that hurt and sometimes sideline you. Then again, employers probably wouldn't hire you if they knew that, right?

The fact is, many people at work (peers and bosses) lack patience when it comes to illnesses. They may have an especially low tolerance for "silly old headaches." (How bad can they be?) They may think that you're a slacker and gossip about your moans and groans.

Most migraine sufferers try to work around their headaches, but they remain misunderstood and their incomes and productivity still suffer. The unemployment rate for those with severe migraines is extremely high.

Migraine sufferers will often freely admit that they need help in handling work situations and quandaries, from dealing with unsympathetic attitudes to making sure that their worker bee profile doesn't suffer.

Migraineurs can be excellent employees, top-notch supervisors, and terrific entrepreneurs and CEOs. Just stay the course — and handle the migraine downside with confidence. Enter your workplace equipped with migraine remedies and surefire survival skills.

Minimizing Migraine's Impact at Work

Migraines can make it hard (but not impossible) to be a shining example of a top-notch work ethic. If you have migraines on a regular or semi-regular basis, you most likely call in sick occasionally, retreat to a dark office to recuperate for a couple of hours, or leave the office early because you're suffering too much to work.

Sure, you hate work absences and downtime, but you also don't like the idea of going to work when you're operating at half-mast. You can't do the quality work that you do when you're up to speed. When you have a migraine, your brain is sputtering and your concentration is faulty.

Still, you want to be perceived as the professional you are. So try to abide by these six critical workplace rules for migraineurs:

- ✔ **Be up front about your migraines.** Let your employer know that you experience migraines and that you have the situation covered — you have effective medication and relaxation techniques, for example. Reassure your supervisor that headaches haven't made you unproductive or unpredictable in the past, and they won't in the future, either. You may find that many employers are understanding and perfectly willing to work with you.

  If your employer seems skeptical when you reveal your headache malady, give him a letter from your doctor that validates your migraine problem and states that it should not hamper your ability to handle your workload. Use this moment to point out that you like your job and don't want anyone to interpret your calling in sick occasionally as an attempt to avoid responsibility or a sign of job burnout.

- ✔ **Know when to clam up around co-workers or clients.** It's important to know when it is or isn't okay to say what's bothering you (the headache). Most of the time, you should keep your pain to yourself.

- ✔ **Avoid the temptation to unload.** Don't reveal more than people want to know. And remember, few people want to know much about your health predicaments or anyone else's.

- ✔ **Accept the inevitable backlash.** Figure out the best way to handle the reactions of migraine-free colleagues and supervisors who don't understand why headache pain sometimes makes you leave work (or stay home from work altogether).

- ✔ **Do a good job.** If you get behind after missing a day, make up for your lack of production by taking work home. Do anything you can to keep a high profile as a top producer whose work is impeccable.

- ✔ **Don't over-delegate your work.** Sometimes a headache makes you want to hand out your assignments to make sure that they get done on time.

This behavior leaves you open to criticism — "Jack never gets his work done — he always pawns it off on co-workers when he has migraines." Even if you're a supervisor, people quickly tire of your not holding up your end of things (does the word "slacker" sound familiar?).

✔ **Take care of yourself.** Don't delay taking your pain medication. Retreat to a dark office and lie down for an hour or so. And if you don't start feeling better, go home. Just be sure to keep your supervisor abreast of what you're doing. Don't slip out the door like a thief in the night; you have a legitimate illness, and it's nothing to be ashamed of.

Coping with Attitude and Agony

You're experiencing the agony of a migraine, and you're thrown into a lion's den of snarling co-workers and eye-rolling bosses. Nevertheless, you can weather the workplace dilemma with flair.

Survival skills for the office basically boil down to three sticky notes you can post on your brain's gray matter for future reference:

✔ Don't go into the nitty-gritty details (vomiting, nausea, pain) of your migraine. (No one really wants to know.)

✔ Don't dramatize your situation. (Go there, and you may become the latest office gossip.)

✔ Don't be fazed by smirking co-workers. (Some people won't believe that you're hurting, but what difference does that make?)

Responding to "how are you doing" questions

Here's the deal: People you work with — those right alongside you and those who are your bosses — may indeed ask how you're feeling. But — and here's the real rub — they don't *really* want to know.

Yes, they care that you're hurting. But most people will get bored in a heartbeat if you supply any of the gory details (pain level, nausea, starry visuals, and so on).

Co-workers are usually just being polite when they ask how your headache is. If you were to translate what they're actually thinking but wouldn't dare say, it would probably sound something like this: "Gosh, I hope Sam is back up to speed by tomorrow, because we have a big project due, and I don't want to have to do his work."

Setting the record straight

We know a graphic artist who began having migraine headaches at age 20. After a couple of years of unsuccessfully treating his headaches with over-the-counter medications, his doctor diagnosed him with migraines. The diagnosis spurred him to eliminate some food triggers, and the doctor tried him on several medications until he found a drug that worked. So he managed to lasso and hogtie his problem long ago, but now he had a new headache-related work problem. His cubicle-mate was driving him nuts with comments about stress. She'd say such things as, "You need to cheer up. Stress is what's giving you headaches."

Finally, the guy just had to set the record straight: "I'm not overstressed. I have no problems meeting deadlines or turning out my work. Stress sometimes contributes to setting off a migraine, but it usually takes more than just stress to get a migraine. You have to have an inherited tendency, and eat something or smell something that triggers a headache, combined, perhaps, with stress. So, stress alone can't do it."

Way more than his cubicle-mate wanted to know, for sure. But his outburst put an end to the lectures. In other words, if someone at work, whom you can't escape, is driving you nuts with migraine myths, strike a pose and speak up. You live with migraines, so you certainly know more about it than they do!

Follow the golden rule of the workplace when it comes to any illness: If someone asks how you're feeling, thank that individual for his concern and keep your response short and sweet. Resist the temptation to unload your burden — save that for a loved one who has to listen. As one Houston real-estate mogul likes to tell her employees, the only right answer to the question "how are you?" is "terrific!"

Keep your response short, but be honest about what's wrong with you. It's okay for people to know that you have migraines — in fact, it's probably best. Otherwise, someone may see you taking medication and start the rumor mill grinding — "He's definitely on drugs. I saw him taking something!" Get a jump on the situation and admit that you have migraines. It's not like they're contagious!

Avoiding theatrics

Sometimes the pain of a migraine is enough to inspire some major theatrics. You may suddenly wax eloquent about the misery caused by your migraine: "Yes, I hurt! I'd love to tell you the depth and breadth of my migraine pain!" Don't go there. Make sure that you avoid any theatrics whatsoever.

In the workplace, playing up your pain usually comes back to haunt you. Far better to stay low-key and do what you need to do. Go lie down somewhere until you feel better, take your pain medication, or simply head for home if it's the only thing that will do the trick. If you need to lie down somewhere, be sure to tell your supervisor — don't just do it without clearing it first.

Most importantly, instead of being dramatic, do something! Take a medication that will help you get back to The Land of The Productive Workers very quickly.

Sloughing off smirkers

You may have trouble with the attitudes of co-workers and supervisors who are suspicious of all kinds of things, such as your leaving work early, taking trips to the restroom to vomit, getting uncharacteristically quiet when you feel bad, and taking refuge in a vacant office to lie down. Remember, what makes total sense to you may look like neurotic behavior to others.

Sure, some people may look at you funny when you announce that you're leaving work to go home and nurse a migraine. Some may even tell you to "get tough" and hint that you're a wimp. Others will be sympathetic.

The point is, you can't change other people's feelings. Don't think that you're going to shape up your colleagues' attitudes or teach them about migraines. They don't get it — and that's okay. You have to live and get along.

Furthermore, if you try to stick up for yourself when you're feeling bad, the high emotion can make your head hurt worse or make you respond irrationally. Just give their nastiness a "whatever," and be on your way.

Handling those moments of feeling misunderstood

On rough days filled with hardhearted responses to your migraines, remind yourself that people are discriminated against in the workplace every single day for all kinds of things, not just headaches.

One man tells of having to leave work early one day in order to take his sick five-year-old to the doctor and hearing his supervisor yell in the hall, "I'm never hiring anyone with kids again!" Instead of trying to respond to the bully boss, he just left the office, did what he needed to do, and came back the next day without a word about the incident.

Remember, you're probably not going to change your supervisor's existing prejudices. And unless you're miserable enough to look for another job, you need to cope effectively. The one thing you can do, however, is tuck away the info about your boss's behavior as a note to yourself: "If I'm the boss someday, I'll make a point of being compassionate to employees' problems."

If your supervisor is the one giving you flak, rest assured that firing you for a chronic illness isn't going to fly with the workforce commission (unless you're missing work all the time).

Be aware that some people use migraines as an excuse to miss work frequently. You don't want to be a member of that group! Stay home to nurse a headache only when it's absolutely necessary.

Staying in a Positive Self-Image Place on Migraine Days

Sure, you know how to count your blessings. Ever since you first discovered that you were cursed with head-stabbing horrors, you learned to say "at least it's not something more serious" or "well, I'm alive, sort of. . . ."

At the same time, though, maintaining a strong work profile can be tough on the days you're toting a basket full of concrete on your head (at least, that's the way it feels).

Making sure you're understood

You can do several things to make sure that your migraine philosophy is understood. Here are some helpful tips for conveying your philosophy effectively:

- **Tell the truth.** The first time you have to leave work early or call in sick because of a migraine, explain to your supervisor that you get a headache about once a month (or however often you get migraines), and promise to make sure that the drawback won't affect how you handle your workload or the quality of your work.

- **Be matter-of-fact, not sappy.** When you need to take off work or ask for an extended deadline, state your case clearly and succinctly. You're not asking for a major raise. You're only asking for the same consideration that any employee should get.

- **Be a bit of a stoic.** Make sure that you let your boss know that you will not let a little twinge of migraine make you a flight risk. It takes a really bad headache to send you packing. Explain that you prefer to stay at work and do your job — going home is a last-resort for a headache that makes it impossible for you to perform.

- **Show your confidence.** Don't grovel. Never act as if your employer is doing you a huge favor by keeping you on the payroll. You're there to earn your keep, and that's what you do.

✔ **Don't act like you expect special treatment.** Make it abundantly clear that you will always do your work — what's on your job description and more. Volunteer for extra tasks, and be an exemplary employee (a good idea for anyone in the workplace, with or without migraines).

Keeping your chin up no matter how much your head hurts

When you're often afflicted with migraines, maintaining a positive attitude can be a tricky enterprise, especially at work. You don't want to give in to work-related headache despair — even though, at times, it does seem like the cards are stacked against you. You want to find a way to take a survivalist attitude and defuse your frustration.

If you're at work, and you feel too bad to drive home, lie down on a sofa in a vacant office and wait out your migraine attack. Again, you must be sure to get permission from your employer first.

Grabbing a lifeline on an important workday

A stock broker had just landed a primo job. Five months into the stint, he was going strong, finding his footing and taking on extra responsibilities. His boss was having him run meetings. He was also being considered for a promotion — a position in which he would supervise 15 people and interact with top management.

"Things were looking good until one day when I was supposed to give a big presentation to a major client and I got a migraine. I took Advil Migraine, but that wasn't helping, and by noon, I was vomiting, and my head was hammering. I had no idea how I was going to speak and sound like I was making sense at the meeting that afternoon. Things were looking dim, and I was almost giving in to total despair. This would seal my fate — if I bowed out with a headache, of all things, who among this group of men would take me seriously after that?"

Fortunately, he remembered some survival-skill pointers that his father — who was also a migraineur — had mentioned years ago. With the help of the pointers, he was able to reschedule the meeting without annoying anyone or jeopardizing his rising-star status.

"My father told me to proceed with certainty and refrain from making excuses or overexplaining. He said that most people tell too much. Instead, say what you want to do (change a meeting date, in this case) and don't feel like you have to go into great detail or even mention your migraine."

He was able to notify the client two hours in advance (before the client left his office) by sending an e-mail that read: "An unforeseen problem has arisen. Sorry to topple your schedule, but could we reschedule the meeting, at your convenience, of course." They wound up meeting a week later. He got the client on board, and no one ever even knew (or cared) why the date of the meeting was changed.

The following tips can help you handle workplace snafus without missing a beat and reduce the likelihood of falling into a headache-despair spiral:

- ✔ **Know when you're being trumped.** Be wary of a co-worker or supervisor who tries to use your headache disability as a trump card. When someone interrupts you — "Well, I'll take over because you're probably half-steam today with that migraine" — don't hand over the reins to the steamroller. Go ahead and complete your statement, and make sure that you don't let the end of your sentence trail off into uncertainty.

- ✔ **Avoid putting too much information on the table.** In many instances, you don't need to alert people that you're off your game. Avoid statements like: "Don't mind me — I know I sound vague, but I have this awful headache. . . ."

- ✔ **Reduce your anxiousness by coming up with a game plan.** Sketch out in advance what you'll do on headache days. Decide how much you can handle on a workday when your head is hurting, and do just that. Save your most difficult and mind-bending projects for days when you're going full-tilt.

Don't wear blinders! Recognize when you're not being effective or your messages aren't clear, and take either of these events as a signal that you may need to go home and get to feeling better before you try to continue your work. If you're so off-kilter that you're not even making sense anymore, you only make yourself look ridiculous by sticking around.

If you're constantly getting upset because your migraines cause you to miss work so often, you need to see your doctor to discuss possibly starting preventive migraine medication. You may want to consider looking for a job that is less structured, or one that you can do as a contractor or freelancer. If you're slowed by a headache at a less structured job, you can make up for lost time later when you're feeling better, as long as you turn out the work by the agreed-upon date.

Working with Periods of Disability

The truth is, some people with chronic migraines face periods of disability — possibly a few days a week every month. So your best bet is to come up with a strategy for handling these periods of disability — if they occur.

You already know if you're debilitated by your headaches — or if your loved one faces periods of disability because of migraines. You may live in fear that the time will come when headaches will disrupt your ability to earn a living. A migraine not only causes physical pain, but it can impair your mental and physical functioning, which can make it disabling.

Applying for disability benefits can be a long and drawn-out affair. You also have to struggle with the challenge of having a disability that can't be quantified via specific diagnostic tests. Currently, Congress is investigating the possibility of adding medical evaluation criteria for migraines to Title II of the Americans With Disabilities Act.

No one should treat you unfairly because you have migraines. If you're capable of doing your job satisfactorily, no one can fire you just because you have migraines. You, as a migraine sufferer, have rights under the Americans With Disabilities Act. At the same time, though, you have to accept the responsibility of doing everything you can to cope successfully with your headaches so that you can work.

In most cases, migraine sufferers find a migraine medication that works well. Effective medications can help you avoid missing work as often.

How do you know if your migraines qualify as a disability? According to the disability rules, you must have a physical and/or mental problem that keeps you from working for at least 12 months or is terminal (will result in death). It's very unlikely that migraines will fit this description — they aren't terminal, and headaches shouldn't disable anyone for a year. But if you want to find out if you're eligible for disability payments, call the National Social Security office at 1-800-772-1213. You can file a claim at your local Social Security office. If necessary, take along a family member or friend to help you.

When you place your call or go to the Social Security office, have the following information handy:

- ✔ Social Security card (or number)

- ✔ Your medical records (Contact your doctor to get copies of these. List any abnormal tests, all medicines, and all treatments.)

- ✔ A list of all doctors and clinics that have evaluated and treated you (You'll need phone numbers, addresses, and fax numbers.)

- ✔ A list of the medications you're currently taking

- ✔ A work resume (If you don't have a resume, make a list of your jobs since high school: include names of companies you worked for, each supervisor's name, your jobs performed, and the years you were there.)

You can find information on the disability programs the U.S. government offers at the Social Security Administration Web site (www.socialsecurity.gov). Filing a claim is no swift process, but if you're approved, the money will be helpful if you're disabled.

Your Social Security office refers your claim and all related information to a state agency that will determine whether you're eligible for disability benefits.

A board of reviewers will look over your file and notify you if additional information and medical testing are required. After the review board has everything in hand, it'll make a final determination and let you know whether your claim was approved. If it is approved, the review board will tell you the amount of money you receive and when payments should begin.

If you get a thumbs down on your claim, you can appeal the decision. The office that issued the refusal can tell you how to file an appeal.

Many large companies have disability benefits. If your company offers disability benefits, and you're rendered disabled by your migraines, you may be granted an early retirement with disability pay.

If you have questions about your rights as a migraineur in the workplace, contact the Migraine Awareness Group: A National Understanding for Migraineurs (MAGNUM), a group that educates people about migraine, disseminates information, and works with the government on migraine disability, insurance, and research issues. You can find MAGNUM on the Internet at www.migraines.org.

Today, with numerous migraine medications available that can work wonders for headache sufferers, the likelihood of your suffering a permanent disability from migraines is practically nil.

Handling absences with dependability and competence is your best bet for workplace survival. Also, celebrate the fact that you live in an era when you have access to many excellent migraine remedies that can help you live a normal life.

Chapter 17

Handling Your Home Life

*I*s your family getting cheated because they live with a migraine sufferer whose on-again, off-again ways often lead to frustration and disappointment? You may harbor some fear about the deterioration of your home life due to your headache problems.

But despite your headaches, you can still be an amazing parent, mate, and person. Never doubt it. No matter how frequent or severe your headaches, your home absolutely doesn't have to be the Dark Dungeon of Migraine Suffering. On the contrary, with support and help from family members, you can handle a dreary health condition with optimism and finesse.

It's important, of course, to use tender loving care in dealing with the confusion and hurt of your children when they question why you can't be at their soccer playoffs, choir concert, or graduation. Also, patiently and gently help your mate come to an understanding of what it's like to live with a chronic illness.

If you have a relative whose negative attitude grates on your nerves, you can develop a set of responses to handle her rude comments. These lines will come in handy, especially if The Annoying One starts spouting off when you're suffering the pain of a migraine.

Try to get a grip on your home life early in your headache history. Apply tact and strong coping skills. If you want to scream because family members are complaining about your cancellations of trips, evenings out, and events, remember that their interest in having you on board for everything is a compliment — they enjoy your company! Let them know how very much you want to be involved, and how you plan to do everything you can to ensure that you're a frequent flyer when it comes to family outings.

Giving Cues to Loved Ones

Your household ambiance can be everything you want it to be with some creative thought and ready-for-sick-days planning.

If you're like many migraine sufferers, you may fall deep down into poor-me despair — "I'm always disappointing people!" — when you realize that your family has trouble understanding migraines and coping with the effects migraines have on their lives.

Here are some tips for keeping your home relationships healthy:

✔ **Educate your family.** It's up to you to inform those you love about migraines and dispel myths and misconceptions. Point them to Web sites (see Chapter 9) that offer information on migraines and how to cope with them. Explain the hereditary aspect of migraines.

You may want to show your loved ones pictures that some migraineurs have drawn to show how their pain feels. You can find some pictures on the MAGNUM (Migraine Awareness Group: A National Understanding for Migraines) Web site at www.migraines.org. These graphic illustrations of the horror of migraine misery may convey the message far better than your words can.

✔ **Let people know what you need from them.** Express your needs clearly. Remember that your loved ones aren't mind readers.

✔ **Give ample reassurance.** Clarify that a headache isn't something you can predict or anything they can cause. Relatives may jump to the wrong conclusions when you say that you have a headache: "Are our kids making too much noise? Do you want us to send them outside?" Or, if you cancel on a family gathering, family members may assume that you don't want to be there. It's your job to let them know that your headache is to blame, not anything else.

Expressing what you need

When it comes to dealing with your migraines, you probably already know two things quite well: what family members can do to help during your headache suffering, and what you wish they wouldn't do. Perhaps you find yourself lying in bed, wishing that someone would turn down the loud TV, make the dog stop barking, or stop the squabbling.

Wishes don't enlighten others unless they're expressed.

Say clearly and kindly what you want more of and what you want less of: "I love it when you offer to bring me something to drink," or "It bothers me when you tell me 'oh, cheer up and you'll feel better.' If it were that easy, don't you think I'd do it?"

Typically, family members who know how to help the migraineur, even in very small ways, tend to feel a reduced sense of frustration and helplessness. No one likes seeing a loved one experience pain. It feels even worse if you can do nothing but stand by and feel impotent.

Don't hesitate to turn to a family counselor if your family members grow increasingly frustrated and angry by your headaches. They may feel resentful of the burden your migraines impose on the family. Having this problem unresolved is detrimental to the family unit.

Getting a handle on your emotions

You feel a headache coming on, so of course you want to zap it if you can. But if your first attempt fails, go to Plan B — create a day's agenda that's doable for you. On migraine days, do what you can to smooth your own emotional path.

For example, if you feel that your migraines are misunderstood by a certain family member, try to limit your time with that person on the day you have a migraine. Interact primarily with people who have empathy for your situation and aren't going to crank up your pain level with their questions and criticisms.

You may also fear that being in pain will make you curt or temperamental with your loved ones, or that your kids won't have much fun if you're not around to step up to the plate as recreation director.

Keep in mind that you may not like the way you feel and act during the drugged aftermath of a migraine anymore than you do during its onset. You may be edgy, irritable, easily agitated, and impatient.

Replace your negative mind script with positive thoughts. Every time a negative thought pops into your brain, replace it with one that's more productive and optimistic. Consider the following negative statements and their possible replacements:

- ✔ "I constantly let everybody down."

    Replace with "I often meet people's needs when I'm feeling good, which is most of the time."

- ✔ "My kids are going to wish they had another mom."

    Replace with "My kids may wish I didn't have migraines, but they're glad I'm their mom."

✔ "I bet my husband wishes he hadn't married such a lame headache loser."

Replace with "My husband loves me and wishes I didn't have headache pain, but we have lots of good times together. No one is healthy all the time."

✔ "I hate to ask people to do things for me — I think I'm imposing on them."

Replace with "I do things for my family, and they probably don't mind helping me out."

✔ "I want to bite my mate's head off when she says 'cheer up.'"

Replace with "I'm going to think before I speak, because I know it's hard for my mate to understand what I'm going through, and I'm sure she means well."

Feeling guilty or bad about yourself doesn't help anyone — especially you.

Making Your Mate an Advocate

If you're married, getting your mate to be your health advocate may be as simple as letting her know what you need from her. This approach is something she can get her teeth into — much more appealing than addressing the baffling confusion she may feel when faced with your occasional retreat into the hellishness of a migraine.

Line up your mate as your number-one supporter. Reassure her on those days when you have to pull back from sexual activity because your head is hurting. With her on your team, you'll feel better just knowing that you have an empathetic partner with you in the pain trenches.

Recruiting a best buddy for the migraine wars

Freely admit to your mate your emotional distress over having migraines. And tell your mate what she can do to help you get through the rough times more smoothly. (You can find some tips in Chapter 25.)

Essentially, you want to feel like she's on your team, which means that she's ready to do the following when you have a headache:

✔ Keep the home's noise level down as much as possible

✔ Respect your inability to function fully

✔ Resist trying to engage you in conversations or send you on errands

✔ Take care of anything that comes up that requires an immediate response or decision

✔ Act as a buffer zone and go-between by filling in other household members on how bad your headache is

Explaining "not tonight, honey, I have a headache"

If you have migraines, any kind of movement or exertion may make your headache worse. When you have a migraine, you probably can't imagine wanting to have sex or understand why your mate would want to have sex with someone who's so obviously sick and out of it. You may think, "Why can't she just understand how awful I feel. Do I *look* sexy right now?"

Frankly, you expect some grown-up understanding from your mate. But when the thorny issue of sex is on the table, many an otherwise understanding partner may seem irrational and demanding.

It's better to deal with the sex-or-no-sex issue on a day when you don't have a headache. Don't wait until you have a migraine to discuss the sex question.

Being Realistic about Your Children's Reactions

As a migraineur, you have probably felt the strain of being the Cinderella who was left behind while everyone else went to the ball. Not being able to participate in activities that you were looking forward to with relish is enough to make you blue, no doubt about it. The cancellations. The postponements. The disappointments. It's tough dealing with your own feelings of frustration and resentment.

If you're a migraineur with kids, the absolute worst part of dealing with migraines is the impact that they can have on your children. You may worry about your children having to live in a household that goes on quiet lockdown whenever you get a headache. Unable to show their zestful youthfulness, your children may resent the many restrictions and wonder why their mom or dad can't be normal like other parents — or at least that's what you may fear.

To improve your relationship with your children, you can lead them to a greater understanding of the situation and the fact that you hurt, and find ways to make up for the days when you can't be 100-percent vital and active.

Making some migraine rules for your kids

First, draw your children close. Don't shut them out. Let them know how migraines make you feel, and that you don't like being out of commission and apart from them, and reassure them that they're not to blame for your migraines. When discussing migraines with the very young, you can rub your head and inform them that it hurts. The word "hurts" is a familiar word, so they should have some vague idea of what you mean.

The following tips can help keep your parent-child bond strong and intact:

- ✔ **Set up boundaries for headache times.** Make clear rules about noise levels and play areas that are to be observed during those times when you're suffering with a headache. Discuss these rules in a family meeting when you're not sick. Explain that the rules will help you feel better sooner.

- ✔ **Don't expect young children to understand your migraines.** Your children may not understand that you're sick. They may be confused by your changeable self, and that's just normal for youngsters.

- ✔ **Ask your children to accept your down times.** "If you will try to understand me when I'm not at my best, or when I'm feeling a little grumpy or moody, I'll understand when you're in a bad mood."

- ✔ **Explain what's going on.** Tell your children that you're ill and you're certainly not just trying to get away from them by hiding in your bedroom.

- ✔ **Keep things as routine as possible.** Make a point of doing everyday things, such as giving goodnight kisses and morning hugs, and saying "I love you," even when you're down and out with a headache.

Respecting kids' priorities

Try to give priority to the activities that are important to your children and that you can manage to do even when you're sidelined with a migraine.

Don't beat yourself up about the things you're unable to do. Instead, pat yourself on the back for managing to rally for a few special moments during your headache.

Here are some ways you can show that you respect your children's priorities even when you're sick with a migraine:

- ✔ **Make a cameo appearance.** If your daughter's favorite part of the day is her bath or tuck-in time, try to show up for it, even if it's just for a brief moment.

- ✔ **Don't make your child feel bad for being disappointed.** When you're sick in bed, your child *does* feel bummed, and your guilt-tripping her about natural feelings will only make matters worse. Sure, she may feel let down, but if you're really with her when you're headache-free, she's still going to thrive.

- ✔ **Comfort a sad child.** If your child cries for you when you're out of commission, offer comfort — a kiss, a hug, or a few whispered words. She may miss you and want you back on board, so reassure her that you'll be better soon (probably tomorrow morning). You may also want to offer to participate in a special activity when you're feeling better: "We can look forward to breakfast together — I'll even make you dog-shaped pancakes."

- ✔ **Stay in view so that you don't become a phantom parent.** The migraineur who lies in a dark room may look very scary to a young child. You may appear to be a different person from the cheery, smiling parent she knows, and this can be unsettling.

Don't hesitate to smile and hug your child even when you have a blazing headache. You don't have to talk much — just show that you're still the same old loving you.

Handling the Negative Attitudes of Family Members

Go ahead and own the truth. Yes, your headaches sometimes mess up family fun, but so what. People develop character when everything in their lives isn't perfect every single day.

At the same time, you shouldn't be surprised if you get negative comments from time to time. Again, so what. Let people feel the way they do. You can't change their thinking.

From the minds of babes

Every child is affected differently by living with a parent who has debilitating migraines. And each child will remember her feelings in her own way. So it's important to be reassuring and promote an understanding of the times when you're not functioning well. If you practice good communication, your child will have a better grasp of your illness and find it less frightening.

The daughter of a migraineur named Clinton Shirley relates her memories of growing up with a headache dad: "My father had frequent migraines, and for each of us kids, something different stood out in our memories about his being sick. I remember my dad's face looking gray, and seeing him lying in bed or hearing him vomiting. My mother made us tiptoe around the house, and I was afraid he was going to die."

Her brother: "I remember trips having to be canceled and missing out on doing things. It was hard to make a plan because we kids couldn't drive, and our mother didn't drive on freeways. One time Dad was supposed to take a group of kids to a movie and he got a headache, so that was the end of that plan."

Her older sister: "I remember how Daddy suffered in silence and tried not to burden anyone with his pain. He would come home from work early and sit in his chair and stay very quiet. He wasn't even grouchy with us. I felt sad for him."

Her dad: "I think of all the time I lost, being sick — time when I couldn't be productive or do things with my wife and children."

At age 60, though, her father finally saw his headaches decrease in severity and frequency, exactly what one doctor had said would happen with aging.

Today, at 83, Clinton Shirley is a healthy and joyful senior citizen who has one mild-to-moderate migraine once every two or three months — usually after a being exposed to bright sunlight on fishing trips. He's a perfect example of someone for whom the triptan drugs for migraines (or a preventive migraine medication) would have granted a very different life, with far less downtime.

But, you can wage a worthy comeback that puts a positive face even on headaches: "Hey, who's better equipped to appreciate being pain-free than a person who suffers migraines? I never take good health for granted."

If you're accused of playing up your pain to get sympathy, don't try to win the debate. Don't fret about it. Some people get their kicks from being critics.

Have a clear and present strategy for keeping your family from imploding because of your migraines. Don't let headaches minimize your role as mother, father, sister, or brother. During headache-free periods, stay just as vivid and viable and active as you want to be. Avoid your headache triggers, follow your migraine-management plan, and take your meds properly.

And don't guilt-trip yourself if and when a headache hits and pulls you out of the game. With any luck, your life will soon be humming along again, right on schedule.

Part VI

Managing Special-Situation Migraines

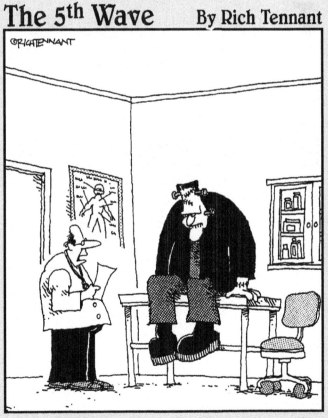

The 5th Wave   By Rich Tennant

"We've tried adjusting your diet, and prescribing medication for your migraines. Now, let's try loosening some of those bolts and see if that does anything."

In this part . . .

This part tells you what you've long suspected — migraines are chameleons, which is exactly what makes them such scoundrels to treat. They can be erratic (on a good day). Your best bet, as a smooth and savvy migraineur, is to get up-close and personal with your own strain of migraines so that you can become an expert at managing them.

Part VI covers the hammering that hurts children's noggins; the hormonal hullabaloos staged in female heads; the migraine mischief that plagues seniors; stress-related headaches; sex migraines; and the dangerous headaches that require a trip to the emergency room.

Chapter 18

Spotting the Dangerous Headache

*W*hether you're new to migraines, or you've had them for 20 years, you need to be familiar with the symptoms that should send you scurrying to the emergency room. A horrible headache can be a sign of some very serious medical problems. As a migraineur, you may be at a disadvantage in recognizing these danger signs as a problem, because you naturally just think, "Oh wow, another bad headache!"

You should know what's different about a dangerous headache and be prepared to handle one. For most headache sufferers, setting up a game plan for the time when you may have a seriously awful migraine is a great idea. You probably won't need to use your game plan, but the knowledge may come in handy if you ever experience that most unbelievable of all headaches.

Paying Attention to First-Ever or Worst-Ever Headaches

First-ever and *worst-ever* are two key terms to remember when assessing whether a gut-wrenching headache should send you rushing to the emergency room. You notice increased pain, more frequent headaches, or a change in your headache type. Then you get a really awful headache. Ask yourself these questions: "Is this my first-ever such headache? Is this my worst-ever headache?" If you answer yes to either question, scurry to the nearest emergency room, or get someone to take you if you feel like you're too sick to drive.

In truth, the likelihood that you have a serious medical problem is very slim. Very rarely does a bad headache actually signal an awful situation in your body. Furthermore, if something is amiss in your brain, a headache probably won't be the lone symptom. Chances are, you'll have several red flags waving "dangerous curves ahead."

Spotting ER-Worthy Red Flags

Severe headaches are not to be taken lightly. Don't fool around with any of the following symptoms, because they're signs that you need immediate medical attention:

- At age 50 (or older), you start having bad headaches.
- Your headaches are becoming more painful and more frequent.
- Your headache is easily the worst of your life.
- You have sudden, piercing pain. (It may be a cluster headache, but you can't assume that it is unless you've been evaluated by a doctor.)
- You have an existing medical problem, such as cancer, AIDS, diabetes, or high blood pressure.
- You have bad headaches that are most severe when you wake up in the morning, and are accompanied by vomiting, seizures, weakness, clumsiness, and/or personality changes.

  The fear with these symptoms is that you may have a brain tumor.
- You have a severe migraine attack that lasts more than 72 hours, and you may be vomiting and dehydrated.

  These symptoms may signal status migrainosus (see Chapter 4). They should be treated as a medical emergency.
- Your headaches get worse when you exert yourself in some way, such as with exercise or sex.

  You probably have a migraine, but if you're experiencing this kind of headache for the first time, or if you've never been evaluated for these headaches, seek medical attention, because it may be a ruptured brain aneurysm.
- Your headache is accompanied by odd symptoms, such as loss of consciousness, difficulty talking or moving, weakness in your arm(s) or leg(s), difficulty walking, loss of vision, or abnormal eye movements.
- Your headache is accompanied by a fever, a stiff neck, or a rash.

  A headache that's associated with some of these symptoms can be caused by an intracranial infection such as meningitis, encephalitis, or a brain abscess. Vomiting and/or sensitivity to light often occur, but they are also experienced with migraine.

✔ You have headaches after (or within several weeks of) a head injury or whiplash.

   This symptom can be a sign of concussion, subdural hematoma, or post-traumatic headache.

✔ You have a family history of brain aneurysms, and you're starting to have headaches.

✔ You feel confused, exhausted, or lightheaded, or you notice (or someone tells you) that your speech and/or movement are abnormal.

✔ You have memory loss and blurred vision along with a headache.

✔ You have severe pain near the base of your skull in the back of your head, or above your eye or ear.

   If this headache is accompanied by neurological problems (such as slurred speech, muscle weakness, double vision, fainting, or partial or total blindness), it may be a basilar migraine, which can lead to a transient ischemic attack (TIA) or stroke. (*Transient ischemic attacks* are caused by a disruption of blood flow to the brain and are sometimes called warning strokes or mini-strokes — they result in temporary neurological dysfunction.)

   Women who use birth control pills, smoke, and have high blood pressure are at higher risk for stroke associated with migraine.

A doctor will want to check you out if you show any of these red-flag symptoms, but remember, you probably *aren't* suffering from a serious health condition. Still, you may go in for an MRI or CT scan (see Chapter 6) to rule out serious problems. In the case of a brain tumor or hemorrhage, it would be quite out of the ordinary for a headache to be the only symptom.

Detecting what's different

You need to be able to detect what's different about a headache that may point to a serious condition so that you'll know when you need a medical evaluation. The simple rule is to think trouble in either of the following situations:

✔ Your headache is unlike anything you have experienced in the past (more painful, more intense, more sudden, and so on).

✔ You're older than 50 and you're having your first awful headache.

It's important to remember that a thunderclap-like head pain has many possible causes — from migraine to certain eye disorders to stroke — so it's important to have it checked out right away.

Handling the groundswell of trouble

If you have a headache that's sudden, severe, and persistent, you should seek medical attention as soon as possible.

A headache accompanied by symptoms such as dizziness, weakness on one side of the body, numbness in any part of your body, staggering, slurred speech, droopiness on one side of your face, or breathing difficulties may indicate a serious problem such as a stroke.

A high-voltage thunderclap-type headache accompanied by a stiff neck, confusion, nausea and vomiting, sensitivity to light, and/or decreased consciousness may be a sign of bleeding in the brain.

If you suspect trouble, an immediate trip to the ER is in order! At the hospital, your doctor may decide that you need surgery, medication, or some other form of treatment. But time is of the essence if you're having a stroke, so don't waste time deliberating about whether to seek help or not. Just do it.

Getting Thee to the ER on Time

The ER doctor's goal is to exclude the presence of life-threatening conditions as soon as possible. He will perform a physical and neurological examination. If the exam is normal, he may not order additional diagnostic tests (depending on your symptoms).

A neurological exam involves a series of simple exercises to test your strength, reflexes, coordination, and sensation. Your doctor may ask questions to asses your short-term memory and mental acuity.

The physical and neurological examinations can usually rule out life-threatening conditions. If the doctor decides that you don't need more tests, he'll help you get rid of your worst-ever headache by giving you medication. (The excruciating pain may make it hard to believe that you don't have something catastrophic, but getting good news is always a relief, nonetheless.)

Basically, your doctor weighs your red-flag symptoms (see "Spotting ER-Worthy Red Flags," earlier in this chapter) and decides whether you need additional tests, such as a CT scan (computerized tomography), MRI (magnetic resonance imaging), or lumbar puncture (spinal tap), to determine what's wrong. (See Chapter 6 for more on these tests.) Usually, tests aren't required to diagnose migraines. Instead, they're used to rule out other problems.

When tests are run because you have a severe headache, the findings are usually normal. However, if you have any red-flag symptoms, it's extremely important and urgent to have them evaluated by a doctor.

Calling wolf one too many times (the ER junkie)

We heard of a man who went to the emergency room with frightening headaches four times before he finally realized that he needed to see a headache specialist and get some medication that would either stop his headaches or help him handle the pain. Over-the-counter (OTC) remedies clearly weren't working for him. When these remedies failed, he got so frantic, he ended up in the ER.

"The ER doctor gave me an injection to stop the horrible headache pain, but told me that what I was using for headache management wasn't optimal — and suggested that I see a headache specialist for evaluation and treatment." He knew that he felt panicky because his headaches were so excruciating. He wasn't sure which symptoms or signs were ER-worthy, and which ones were just the result of another migraine.

After three visits to his headache specialist for evaluation and treatment, Bart had a plan, a prescription medication, and good information about when to go to the ER and how to recognize a migraine. Of course, he didn't intend to end up an ER junkie, but his head pain drove him to desperate measures. Fortunately, he finally got a tip from a doctor that spurred him to take the time to investigate his migraines.

Chapter 19

Let's Hear It for the Girls: Hormonal Migraines

According to the National Women's Health Information Center (U.S. Department of Health and Human Services), 20 million women in the United States have headaches — 9 million of whom suffer debilitating migraines. Compared to men, the prevalence of migraines in women is two to three times higher. The nature of women's migraines is different, as well: They're usually more painful and longer-lasting, they often come with nausea and vomiting, and they typically have fewer visual disturbances (when compared to men's migraines).

Women aged 30 to 45 endure the most migraines. After age 50, most female migraine sufferers see a decrease in the number and severity of headaches. (Who says middle age doesn't have some advantages?)

Half of all women who suffer from migraines report an association between their headaches and their menstrual cycles. Most researchers believe that the ogres behind women's migraine headaches are female hormones — estrogen, in particular. Estrogen affects the functioning of *serotonin,* a neurotransmitter substance (brain messenger) in the nervous system. Basically, when estrogen levels fall, serotonin levels plummet, too, and this often gives rise to migraines. Most migraine sufferers (of both genders) seem to have an inherited condition that makes them ultrasensitive to the effects of serotonin changes.

This chapter will help you find solutions for these hormonal headbangers. Join our Migraine-Busting Gang and discover clues in estrogen/progesterone patterns that can lead you and your doctor to the most effective medications and the most beneficial lifestyle changes for you, no matter what stage of life you're in. If you're pregnant, you need to know which drugs won't hurt the baby in tow. And, if you're 40-plus, you may need info on battling the migraines of menopause. At any rate, get revved up for the challenge, because we're here to tell you that you *can* tame the beast.

Discovering Why So Many Women Are Plagued by Migraines

Because you're female, you're very likely to experience headaches as you bounce along life's long and winding road. Migraines may first hit when you begin having menstrual periods in adolescence. And then your menstrual cycle may force you to tiptoe through the migraine land mines for years. Starting your period can actually kick off decades of vulnerability to migraines.

You may have migraines as big as Texas, or you may have ones that are fairly manageable. Or you may be subject to other varieties of headaches, such as tension headaches, cluster headaches, or sinus headaches, or even headaches that are secondary to a medical condition or injury. (See Chapter 4 for more on these types of headaches.)

Basically, if you do get migraines, the reason is probably one of these:

- ✔ Sudden drops in estrogen and progesterone
- ✔ Progesterone levels are too low
- ✔ Estrogen levels are either too high or too low

The rise and fall of the hormone empire

At the start of your cycle, the two hormones that direct the process — progesterone and estrogen — are at their lowest levels. Gradually, over the next 14 days, estrogen creeps up higher until it reaches a peak around day 15, when you ovulate (prime time for getting pregnant).

You're much less likely to have a migraine during the first part of your cycle, but matters shift quickly after ovulation. Estrogen levels decline for a few days before reaching their next high four or five days before your period starts. Progesterone, which began rising right after ovulation, peaks on about day 23.

The tricky part comes after day 23, when both estrogen and progesterone do a free fall, upsetting the delicate body balance and wreaking havoc in women who are predisposed to migraines.

Your physical response to these hormone swings can complicate the bodily balance — your body reacts to the hormone swings by cranking up its production of prostaglandin, a hormonelike substance that makes you more sensitive to pain. So you may say that the deck is stacked against you, with a trifecta hormone whammy that's not doing you any favors.

Looking for pain relief on the operating table

Watch out! Think a long time before going with the proposal that you may be able to vanquish your migraines via a hysterectomy, thus getting rid of those cumbersome female organs and their accompanying hormone hailstorms. This may not be the best solution; you can end up getting the surgery needlessly. Definitely seek a second opinion if a doctor tells you that a hysterectomy is your best bet.

A California woman tells her poignant tale: "I'm 42, and I get two to three migraines a week. People think you're imagining them, so I feel defective. You go to the emergency room with a headache, and they think you're a drug addict and you're just there to get pills. Also, you're a real low priority in the ER.

"I'm a mess — I'm always in bed. People tell me I'm depressed or stressing, but I don't feel like I'm causing them. I can't go to my son's soccer games, or plan much of anything. I've spent a fortune looking for answers, and I even had a hysterectomy because I was convinced my hormones were the problem; a week later, I had a migraine." Finally, she found Imitrex, a drug that worked for her. "That has made all the difference. I got my life back."

Of course, Imitrex won't work for everyone, but many women find prescription drugs helpful in getting rid of migraines. You keep fighting the good fight until you find something that eliminates the pain. Your female hormones aren't necessarily the key cause for your migraines.

Female hormones can trigger (and perpetuate) migraines by affecting blood flow to the brain. Hormones may also alter the brain's electrical activity. *Serotonin* is considered a catalyst in migraine mischief. It's a message-carrying hormone that's also a migraine trigger in men's headaches. When the hormone hits low levels, it touches off chemical changes that expand blood vessels in the brain and irritate nerves. The distended (puffed-out) vessels are starring players in the Pain Game because they send Big-Hurting-Head pain signals to your brain.

Your migraine pain and other headache symptoms are a result of this complex glitch in usual brain activity. The special system that makes this chain of events a health problem came to you by virtue of your gene pool — you were born female, so you're more likely to have headaches. In addition, you may have a hereditary penchant for migraines.

Many researchers believe that when estrogen falls, so do serotonin levels. And we all know that the female hormone estrogen is to a woman what a Stetson is to a cowboy. With too little of it, you'll have a hitch in your step. Before a woman starts her period, her estrogen levels fall. In the years leading up to menopause *(perimenopause)*, estrogen levels are all over the map. So the serotonin/estrogen connection may explain why lots of women are hit with migraine pain right before their periods — or in the years right before menopause.

One myth is that women have more migraines than men simply because they're the "emotional" gender — they get weepy and upset, and that brings on headaches. Not so. Sure, your head may be pounding when you're upset — make no mistake about it — but it's not because you're high-strung. You have female hormones that sometimes wreak havoc with your brain's messenger troops — and that's a biochemical thing, not a "women's issue."

Physicians once believed that women, because they were so stressed by the rigors of child-rearing, were a bit hysterical in describing their headaches. But over the years, research has borne out the truth — that migraines are no exaggeration or imagined scenario. They're bona-fide biological problems.

Stress does trigger headaches, of course, but migraine folks don't have more stressors than other people in the world. They're subject to the same pitfalls encountered by the rest of the population. (See Chapter 22 for more about the anxiety-migraine link.)

Nevertheless, it's important to get a handle on migraines chiefly because the pain is horrible — and also because you don't want to get pegged as one of the walking wounded. Yes, you have awful headaches. But, no, you won't let your chronic ailment define you as a person. "That woman with the migraines — the one in sales — is always bailing. You can't count on her." The truth is (and you know this from watching the Lifetime Channel or Oprah), using positive self-talk can help you become anyone you want to be. Or, you can use negative self-talk to downgrade yourself ("you lame loser headache girl") and screw up your life. It's all about choices and attitude. See Chapter 16 for migraine strategies for the workplace.

Combating Menstrual Migraines

Sixty percent of female migraine sufferers have migraine headaches during menses as well as at other times during the month, and 14 percent have migraines only during their periods.

Unfortunately, treating menstrual headaches can be tricky, mainly because what works for one woman does not necessarily work for another. So you face a trial-and-error period with various medications to discover what works in your one-of-a-kind body (see Chapters 7 and 8 for info on medications).

Clearly, hormone swings make you super-susceptible to migraines. So get ready to mix it up and become proactive by doing the following:

- ✔ Avoid things that set off your trigger-happy migraines.
- ✔ Make lifestyle changes that improve your overall health picture.
- ✔ Discover the drug that's most effective for you.

PMS woes: Migraines accessorizing monthlies

In some women, migraine headaches come hand in hand with PMS (premenstrual syndrome): A no-good development. And, often, a migraine isn't the only unwanted passenger on the PMS train. Lots of women have scads of PMS symptoms — both physical and emotional. As if crying jags, mood swings, backaches, and bloating aren't disruptive enough, add a screaming migraine to the mix, and you can see why some women feel incapacitated when their period looms near.

The following criteria point to a diagnosis of PMS:

✔ Your symptoms ebb and flow, increasing as your period approaches, and decreasing when the flow starts.

✔ During several consecutive menstrual cycles, you have PMS symptoms (bloating, irritability, mood swings, weight gain, breast tenderness, backaches, binge eating).

✔ The symptoms cut into your normal activities.

Here's a word to the wise for the partner of a PMSing woman who's having menstrual migraines: Please don't tell her that the problem is "all in her head." The pain is in her head, all right, and it's as real as rain — and your suggesting anything else may get you a door-slam, an eye-roll, and a dirty-look. Watch it, bucko!

You can definitely beat those "I am woman, hear me roar" migraines, but you'll probably have to be assertive in letting your healthcare provider know how awful the pain is. Don't let her get away with patting you on the head and giving you an aspirin. (For tips on finding a good migraine doctor, see Chapter 5.)

Sometimes you can prevent menstrual headaches altogether. Your doctor may prescribe a brief course of NSAIDs (non-steroidal anti-inflammatory drugs) to take for several days before menstruation and during the first few days of your period. If it turns out that your migraines can't be staved off in advance, she'll give you a prescription for one of the medications that serve up a knockout punch for the headache when it starts stewing in your head. (See Chapter 8.)

Finding answers in your monthly patterns

You may have migraines that are so in sync with your hormone shifts, that it seems like your migraines and hormones are instant-messaging each other.

You can confirm their communication patterns by taking the first step to finding out what's behind your migraines — keeping a journal of your headaches to see if you can detect any patterns with foods or habits that may be kicking off trouble. Start by trying self-help measures. See if your journaling shows food-to-migraine links, and avoid those foods to see if it helps.

If nothing you try seems to work, set up an appointment with your doctor to discuss your headaches, and prepare a short headache diary to take to her office. Give a rundown on the frequency and length of your headaches, where you are in your menstrual cycle when they occur, the location of the pain, the intensity rating (on a scale of 1 to 10), and the symptoms you experience. You can find out more about headache journals in Chapter 3.

Typically, the woman who's having an *MM (menstrual migraine)* is spared the *aura* — flashing lights or a visual disturbance prior to the pain's onset. The migraines, though, tend to hit in the two-day period right before menstruation or on the first day of flow. Some women report having migraines at midcycle, when they're ovulating — another time you experience a drop in estrogen.

If you're getting the feeling that you're a delicately calibrated instrument who must take good care of herself, that's pretty much the case. And it's especially true if you come equipped with migraine vulnerability, meaning that horrible headaches run in your family (for more information on the inherited headache gene, see Chapter 1).

Staving off the symptoms

Hormone-associated migraines sometimes respond to the same kind of treatment that's used for migraines that don't include the hormone-tribulations. You can manage the kind of migraine that doesn't rock your world with over-the-counter meds or prescription nonsteroidal anti-inflammatories. But for hardcore headaches, your doctor will probably recommend one of the amazing triptans. Triptans revolutionized migraine treatment when they came on the scene, because they can zap headaches in as little as four to six hours. (See Chapters 7 and 8 for more info on medications.)

Essentially, menstrual migraines can be headed off in a variety of ways. Researchers have discovered that

- Oral contraceptives help some women avoid menstrual migraines. Their head-pain problems become less severe and less frequent as the pills even out their hormone imbalances. (But the Pill can also induce headaches in some women. See "Spelling Relief or Trouble: Oral Contraceptives and Migraines," later in this section.)

- Some meds work especially well for tough menstrual migraines. These medications include over-the-counter naproxen sodium (Aleve) and Excedrin Migraine (which contains aspirin, caffeine, and acetaminophen), and prescription drugs such as the triptans Imitrex and Amerge.

- Habitual migraine sufferers (male and female) may benefit from learning stress and relaxation techniques (see Chapter 9).

When preventives don't ward off a migraine attack, other drugs can help you deal with the symptoms. Your doctor may arm you with Midrin or another medication that works well for migraines (see prescription medications in Chapter 8).

You also need to look at the entire lifestyle spectrum of migraine-busting. If you're in your 20s, 30s, or 40s, you'll be facing many years of womanly hormone havoc, so why not get a jump on things? You have to find an approach that works well for you, and that takes a little persistence. You need to find (and avoid) your food triggers, identify exercises that are migraine-friendly, and keep anxiety and other lifestyle bullies in check (see Chapters 11, 12, and 22 for more on these approaches to managing migraines).

Spelling Relief or Trouble: Oral Contraceptives and Migraines

Who would imagine that an innocent little birth control pill could cause a major ruckus in your body? But it's only too true. For some women, taking contraceptive pills makes migraines worse by increasing their frequency and intensity. On the other hand, some gals get some sweet relief when they start on birth control pills; after having battled headaches for years, these women move into a phase where head-pain problems become less severe and less frequent as the pills even up the zoom, zoom, zooming of hormones.

Most women have common migraines (migraine without aura) rather than classic migraines (migraine with aura). (See Chapter 2 for more on auras.) But if you have classic migraines associated with tingling sensations and/or visual disturbances prior to headaches, don't use oral contraceptives — women with classic migraines have an increased risk of stroke. A small risk of stroke is inherent in taking oral contraceptives, anyway.

If you're using an oral contraceptive with a progestin of high or medium *androgenic* (masculinizing, and thus acne-causing) activity, switch to a progestin-containing pill with lower androgenic activity, which is less likely to trigger migraines. You can ask your healthcare provider to give you info on the progestin level of the pills you're currently using. (All oral contraceptives have progestin — it's the synthetic version of the hormone progesterone.)

If your headaches continue to be so awful that they knock you for a loop, your doctor will probably suggest that you try another form of contraception.

By the way, don't take your roommate's birth control pills or pull out a packet of pills you've had for years — especially if you smoke and have high blood pressure. Before getting on the pill, you need clearance from your doctor, because there's a small risk of stroke that goes up in women who are migraine sufferers, smokers, and high-blood-pressure cookers.

If you're on the pill, and you don't want to try another form of birth control (despite the ragged curse of migraines), experiment with controlling headache triggers through diet and lifestyle behaviors. (See the chapters in Part IV for more on prevention and treatment tips.)

Also, the longer you take birth control pills, the better the chance that your migraine frequency will subside.

Speaking of birth control, don't feel guilty when you have to pass on having sex with your honey. "Not tonight, dear, I have a headache" is a cliché all right, but the idea that women use migraines as excuses to avoid sex is a major myth and a bad rap. Faking headaches no doubt happens — but when you really and truly do have a migraine, and the Evil Migraine Force is hammering ten-inch nails into your noggin, does sex actually sound appealing? No way. You fear any sort of movement at all, and you sure as heck want to avoid physical activity, because it only makes the pain worse. (And what is sex if not high-octane physicality?)

So if you're a guy who loves a migraine gal, don't take the occasional brushoff personally. Please. Your sweetie isn't avoiding intimacy with you. She's just blinded by the light (of head-splitting pain). Instead of pouting, give her generous doses of TLC and some quiet, worry-free time to get back to her healthy self.

Tackling Migraines While You're Pregnant — and Afterward

Thank goodness for small favors. While your uterus is enclosing one of the primo small favors (the baby), you get a payoff in the form of no migraines . . . or at least fewer migraines. The time off from migraines is felt in most women who are migraineurs. For the unlucky few, however, migraines get worse, start up for the first time ever, or stay pretty much the same during pregnancy.

Basically, migraine-prone women have two possible windows of relief — when they're pregnant and when they're in their senior years following menopause.

If you have trouble with migraines during pregnancy, don't take any form of medication without checking it out with your doctor first. Don't forget that powerful message telling you that drugs and alcohol creep across the placenta. It's true — and that's why you shouldn't drink alcohol or self-medicate during pregnancy. Your doctor may recommend placing an ice pack on your head, along with taking some acetaminophen. Avoid using aspirin or ibuprofen.

It's important to note that pregnant women shouldn't take Depakote (valproate), because it can cause birth defects.

Chances are, if you still have migraines when you're pregnant, they'll disappear when you're in your second trimester. Around that time, hormone levels even out, morning sickness usually disappears, and your headaches are less hurtful.

Then you have your baby, and all is joyful and stork-filled — until your migraines return in full force; this time they brought along a whole posse to raise the pitch another notch. Again, you can blame it on hormones, especially estrogen, which is rearranging its input now that you're no longer providing direct life-support for a fetus.

You don't need a fortuneteller to clue you into the fact that something's got to give. Some moms have bad migraines after childbirth — occasionally, the worst ones they've ever experienced.

What will give you a little relief? Launch a migraine-busting frenzy, trying medications your doctor prescribes until you find something that works. (See Chapter 8 for more information about prescription medications.)

Ditching the Migraines of Menopause

At some point, you'll probably zero in on some perfectly reliable meds for migraines. These medications allow you to chug along merrily for a number of years — that is, until you edge up on those mysterious and somewhat spooky change-of-life years. At that time, you'll become subject to another hormonal whirlwind — the jittery estrogen of *perimenopause* (the years leading up to menopause).

Sure, midlife is supposed to be ultra-cool. You hit that plateau where you're poised, accomplished, and confident. You have enough attitude to accommodate the needs of a dorm full of 20-year-old girls. But just when you get the professional expertise polished off and the exercise/nutrition thing down pat, you're hit with a total bummer: middle-age migraines. And just when you thought you were going to be appointed commissar of cranial bliss.

Don't worry. Simply crank up your resolve: You have a rendezvous with fate — a future in which headaches are nothing but low-profile, in-your-face gnats that fly around occasionally but are easily handled (swish, swish . . . get away!). And a healthier you will stride the world with migraine empowerment in full bloom.

In the years before and during menopause, you're well aware that hormones dance through your body like heathens, causing or contributing to hot flashes, night sweats, insomnia, and mood swings — to name just a few of the many symptoms of menopause. These rampaging hormones can also trigger migraines. And, if you have your ovaries removed — causing you to experience *surgical menopause* — you're even more likely to see your migraines pump up their agony potential.

For some women, hormone replacement therapy (HRT) is a godsend. It evens out the hormone thing and eliminates the headaches. For other women, though, HRT may kick off headaches or make them worse.

Your doctor or healthcare provider can recommend medication that will help ease your migraine pain, whether you're using hormone replacement or not.

If you've had double the migraine trouble since you've been on HRT, your doctor will probably try changing the type of HRT you take or the delivery method. For example, if you're using a pill, switching to a patch may ease your mind and your migraines. Getting estrogen via the transdermal patch (a patch placed on the stomach or buttocks) often helps female migraineurs get rid of headaches, because it uses lower doses of estrogen.

If you're menopausal or postmenopausal, your doctor may prescribe the migraine fighters known as beta blockers or tricylic antidepressants. Depakote is often the answer for older women who have had *tubal ligation* (a surgical procedure that closes the fallopian tubes to prevent an unfertilized egg from reaching the uterus). See Chapter 8 for more information regarding prescription medications. The meds above are favored for women going through menopause, but they're also used by men and younger women.

At any rate, whether you're 16 or 64, keep your "girls just wanna have fun" banner flying high. No matter what phase of womanhood you're living in, don't let slam-dance head pain get you down. Do what it takes to tame the beast so that you can enjoy being a girl, just like the millions of others from your lace-and-leather gender.

Making the menopause/migraine connection

One 53-year-old woman tells of going through menopause and loving every minute of it: "The last thing I wanted to be during menopause was one of those waif-looking, hand-wringing, vapor-fainting little women. So, two days after my first night of hot flashes, I went to see my gynecologist and walked out of his office with hormone replacement prescription in hand. My hormone crisis was real — still, it was scary to hear that word 'menopause!'

"At any rate, I've been on hormone replacement since I was 45, and I've never felt better in my life; I don't have to worry about getting pregnant. I no longer have the weepy mood dips of menstrual days. The debilitating migraines I had for decades are history. And now I'm just happy and healthy and bewildered that this age can feel so good. Go figure!"

Chapter 20

Helping a Child with Migraines

. . . .

. . . .

*O*ccasionally, infants have headaches (which may be why some babies bang their heads against the end of the crib occasionally). Toddlers get headaches, too — migraines often occur as sidekicks to common infections. Puberty, however, is by far the most common startup time for youngsters' migraines.

Another type of susceptible child is one who has one or both parents with a migraine history. This child sorely needs answers because he's probably looking at a lifelong struggle with head pain. (People can inherit a tendency to have migraines.)

What's a parent to do? If your tyke is otherwise healthy, you just tuck him into bed and hope that he'll sleep off the pain. Occasionally, though, the simple remedies — such as rest and over-the-counter medications (OTCs) — don't provide relief and prescription drugs are necessary. Children may experience vomiting, nausea, and slowed stomach activity as a result of their migraines. Because the latter problem renders medications ineffective, children may benefit most from rectal suppositories for migraines.

Truly, a child who has migraines can still thrive, excel, and become a totally joyful life force — it's your job to lead him in finding (and eliminating) his migraine triggers, getting relief, and handling the social and psychological aspects of being a Headache Kid. (Missing lots of school, soccer games, dance lessons, and family outings can take a huge toll on a youngster.) Yes, migraines can be a big pain, but in this chapter, we show you how to make sure that the apple of your eye doesn't become a side dish to the main course of life.

Recognizing the Signs

An especially troubling aspect of children's migraines is that they usually go undiagnosed. Even though you're a migraineur yourself, the symptoms your child has may be just different enough that you don't recognize his headache as a migraine.

Covering kids' symptoms

What trips up even parents who are migraineurs themselves is that kids' migraines act different than the kind adults have. Instead of experiencing the hallmark one-side-of-the-head pain, small fries may often feel two-sided pounding — and their aches may last no more than a few hours, compared to the marathon monstrosities that hit big people's heads. On the other hand, kids — like adult migraine sufferers — can have nausea and vomiting, light sensitivity, and dizziness. Their hands and feet may feel cold, too. Oddest of all, though, is the *abdominal migraine* — an attack of vomiting and stomach pain, sometimes without the headache itself!

If your child used to have a headache once a month or so, and now he's being hit with them more often — such as two or three times a week — seek medical attention as soon as possible. (See "Heading for the hospital," later in this chapter, for more symptoms that require medical attention.) Headaches that increase in number and severity signal that you need a doctor's assessment of the problem.

An artistic diagnosis

Five-year-old Emma woke up with a headache. It was the third time in three weeks. She was cuddled up at the end of her bed with her "blankie" and didn't want to eat. She whimpered and patted her head and said, "My head hurts." Her mother was taking her to the doctor that morning, so she gave her acetaminophen and a glass of water and asked her to draw a picture of how she was feeling. The young child lacked the vocabulary to express the full-tilt badness of her situation, but she certainly drew a terrific picture, with zigzag lines dancing in front of the girl's eyes (showing her visual disturbance), and her hands holding her head on the sides.

After seeing this nice "diagnostic" drawing, the doctor examined Emma and prescribed an appropriate medication that eased her headache pain. Therefore, in dealing with small fry, it's a good idea to come up with an illustration or word game to get a good description, which will, in turn, empower the doctor.

In babies and toddlers, signs of headaches are odd restlessness, lack of appetite, and lots of crying. However, these signs are also symptoms for a wide range of other problems, so have a healthcare provider evaluate your young one to rule out other medical causes.

When your child has recurring headaches but is otherwise healthy, you're probably looking at migraines. A child with frequent and acute headaches is almost always a migraine sufferer. A headache accompanying an illness is usually a migraine.

In childhood, migraine headaches are frequently accompanied by tummy aches, but in a small percentage of kids, migraines occur without the headache. This condition can last hours or days — the child may also report a feeling of spinning or dizziness, and a desire to get away from bright lights. Diagnosing the problem can be difficult, but it's usually a case of eliminating all other possibilities.

Sorting headache types

The most common types of headaches in children are migraines and tension-type headaches. (Tension-type headaches are most often the problem.) Cluster headaches are rare in both children and adults. (If your doctor refers to *acute recurrent headache,* it means that your child is showing a pattern of headaches with intervals that are symptom-free.)

The following list covers these headache types in more detail:

- ✔ **Tension-type headache:** Your child may have tight neck muscles, head or neck pressure, and a dull ache on one or both sides of the head, and he may squint when he's reading or watching TV. This headache probably won't cause vomiting. Displaying these symptoms daily is not unusual.

  Factors that can aggravate or trigger tension-type headaches include bad posture, eyestrain, hunger, head-and-neck disorders, skipping meals, or anxiety over dreaded events (scary tests, parents' fighting or divorce, and so on). Children get relief for these headaches from ibuprofen or acetaminophen. Also, try to figure out if your child is experiencing extreme stress over certain family or school problems, and, if so, seek a resolution.

- ✔ **Migraine headache:** A child may have throbbing pain on one or both sides of the head, which can be accompanied by nausea and/or vomiting, fatigue, dizziness, food cravings, diarrhea, fever, noise or light sensitivity, or visual disturbances (such as seeing flashing lights or having tunnel vision). The pain of a migraine can awaken a child from his sleep. See treatment options in this chapter under "Seeking Treatment."

Migraine headaches with vomiting and stomach pain — or just stomach pain without the head pain — are called *abdominal migraines*. If your child has vomiting and stomach pain, don't try to diagnose the problem yourself (unless you're a doctor). Seek medical attention for your child as soon as possible. Your doctor will want to examine your child and may want to run tests to check for other symptoms and exclude other causes of the stomach pain (such as appendicitis) before making the diagnosis of abdominal migraines.

Exertion migraines, headaches you get during or after physical activity, are also common in kids. Teen girls may experience menstrual migraines and birth-control pill migraines (see Chapter 19). Three rare kinds of migraines found in children are ophthalmoplegic migraines, basilar migraines, and hemiplegic migraines (see Chapter 4).

✔ **Cluster headache:** Your child may complain of severe one-sided pain located around or behind his eye. These headaches usually last about 30 minutes, and can be accompanied by a runny nose and teariness in one eye. Fortunately, cluster headaches are rare in kids. Treatments for cluster headaches in children include triptans, oxygen, steroids, lithium, verapamil, ergotamine, and methysergide.

About half of the migraines that children experience are linked to infections; the other half are often linked to vigorous exercise, menstruation, and/or heredity. Many children who have migraines have a strong family history of migraines.

Teachers, parents, and outside caregivers need to understand migraine symptoms and prevention measures. That way, they can identify the problem early on and get the child treated promptly and effectively. You can share this chapter of *Migraines For Dummies* with your outside caregiver or have them check out the following Web site: www.headaches.org/consumer/educationalmodules/childrensheadache/chhome.html.

Heading for the hospital

The following symptoms signal that you need to take your child to the emergency room as soon as possible:

✔ High fever, bad headache, vomiting, stiff neck, confusion: These are signs of meningitis (bacterial and viral).

✔ Headaches that are getting more severe and occurring more often: This can indicate a serious problem such as a brain tumor and should be investigated as soon as possible.

✔ Sudden, awful head pain and/or weakness and clumsiness: The source of these symptoms can be a tumor, infection, *hematoma* (a collection of blood in the brain from head trauma), or another serious problem.

✔ Headache accompanied by double vision, vomiting, dizziness, loss of balance, slurred speech, lack of coordination, or weakness: These can be signs of the very rare basilar migraines (see Chapter 4) or a serious medical condition. Seek prompt medical evaluation.

Hunting Down and Disarming the Causes and Triggers

Spotting the cause of a child's head pain requires sifting through symptoms of the various types of headaches (see the preceding "Sorting headache types" section) and being a perceptive observer. Unfortunately, you can't expect a very young child to be good at describing what's wrong, so you'll probably have to search for clues in order to make a good call.

When you're thrashing around to uncover the reasons for your child's migraines, look for the usual suspects, which include the following:

✔ Caffeine and foods

✔ Environment

✔ Erratic sleep patterns (getting too much or too little sleep)

✔ Menstruation (and/or birth control pills)

✔ Physical exertion

✔ Skipping meals

✔ Stress or excitement

Observe your child's eating patterns for a week to see if skipped meals may be triggering migraines. To monitor his sleep, set up a chart to keep track of the times he goes to bed and wakes up, for about two weeks. You can also chart the other triggers from the previous list. The following sections tell you how to disarm these triggers.

Resolving organic causes: Infections and diseases

About half the time, kids have migraines because they have a fever and a virus or other infection. In such cases, your doctor treats the infection, and usually, the migraines become history. Headaches can be caused by illnesses such as mumps, measles, ear infections, and, more commonly, upper respiratory infections.

Organic causes of children's headaches range from the common and less serious (fever and viral infections) to the rarer and more serious (brain tumors, meningitis, leukemia, and head trauma).

If the cause isn't one that can be resolved easily (lowering fever or treating infection), you move into the next level of treatment — a treatment program for the disease your child has — or drug therapy (if he's suffering from chronic migraines).

Making sure your child doesn't miss meals

Make sure that your child doesn't miss meals, which often sets the stage for a migraine. Missing meals can be a big problem when you're dealing with a teenager who may feel virtually bulletproof — until a migraine hits.

The following are good ways to curtail the bad habit of meal-skipping:

- ✔ **Buy your child foods he likes for that rushing-out-the-door breakfast.** Good choices include low-fat granola bars, small bags of whole-grain cereals, plain yogurt with fruit mixed in, and low-fat cream cheese on a whole-wheat bagel.

- ✔ **Explain the downside of missed meals.** Tell your child that he'll be less likely to have migraines if he becomes a grazer, consuming a number of small meals (approximately six) throughout the day so that he's never extremely empty.

- ✔ **Talk to your youngster about ways to watch his weight without skipping meals.** Help him understand that a healthy approach to meals has big payoffs: an energetic body and a mind firing on all cylinders.

For more information on diet and nutrition, check out the following Web sites:

- ✔ Cooper Aerobics Center in Dallas, Texas: www.cooperaerobics.com
- ✔ USDA Food and Nutrition Information Center: www.nal.usda.gov/fnic
- ✔ Children Nutrition Research Center: www.bcm.tmc.edu/cnrc
- ✔ Texas Children's Hospital: www.texaschildrens.org

Reining in food villains

To figure out what kinds of non-behavior-related factors kick off your child's headaches, follow these lifestyle-inventory guidelines:

✔ Keep a food diary of what your child eats and drinks, and be sure to include his caffeine intake. (Ask an older child to maintain this diary himself.)

Your child gets caffeine if he drinks tea, coffee or coffee milk (milk-diluted coffee that parents sometimes give their kids), energy drinks, and soft drinks — or if he eats chocolate.

If you discover that he's loading up on migraine-trigger foods, help him make dietary changes. With children, common villains behind migraines are hot dogs, smoked meats, foods with MSG (monosodium glutamate), cheese, nuts, peanut butter, chocolate, caffeine drinks, and some fruits (plums, bananas, and oranges). See other food triggers in Chapter 11.

✔ Pump up your child's consumption of nutritious foods to promote over-all health. Good health is always a boon in migraine-fighting. Offer plenty of healthy foods, and don't keep pointless snacks around the house. No child really needs cake, potato chips, and preservative-filled snack foods. If you don't have junk food around for him to fill up on, he's more likely to develop preferences for foods that provide good nutrition for his growing brain and body. (Plus, you don't need junk food either!)

Eradicating environmental triggers

Indoor and outdoor environments may be rife with annoyances for small-fry headache sufferers. So if you think that your child's headaches are related to allergens, visit your doctor so that he can evaluate your child and prescribe an allergy medication such as Claritin.

Besides the headache, other symptoms that may signal that an environmental bugaboo is giving your child trouble are

✔ Breathing difficulty or asthma

✔ Chronic ear infections

✔ Eye puffiness and dark circles under the eyes

✔ Rashes

✔ Runny nose

✔ Sinusitis

✔ Throat clearing

Naturally, factors other than your child's environment may cause the symptoms above, but allergens should at least be considered. Sometimes a child who has allergy problems is misdiagnosed as having something else, such as a disease or attention deficit disorder.

To determine whether your child is having headaches due to environmental causes, use a journal to track the symptoms, the places they occurred, what he was exposed to in the environment, and so on. By keeping a journal, you may be able to pinpoint the troublemakers. If the problems are in your backyard, at school, at daycare, or in a caregiver's home, take measures to reduce your child's exposure to the allergens that trigger migraines — or do what you can to improve the problem areas.

If your child still seems highly sensitive to environmental allergens even when he's taking allergy medication, you can try cleansing and tweaking his environment. Some common environmental headache triggers that kids may need to avoid (or handle wisely) are weather changes, smoke-filled rooms, places with strong odors or vapors, dusty outings, pets, and flickering or fluorescent lights.

Check for possible headache-causing odors or allergens in your child's bedroom or your home at large. Beware of stuffed toys, pillows, and blankets: all of these can be havens for allergens. (See Chapter 13 for more on environmental triggers.) Dust allergies are also a common cause of headaches in some people. Unfortunately, allergic folks may have reactions to dust that lurks all over the place — in linens, drapes, and mattresses.

If you can, get rid of the environmental trigger that bothers your child — or show him how to avoid it. On the other hand, if he's stuck in the presence of one that's unavoidable (something at school), let him know how to relax and use imagery to reduce his stress (Chapter 7 includes nondrug remedies). If necessary, your child may need to take an over-the-counter medicine when a headache starts bothering him.

If you want to know specifically what your child is allergic to, take him to an allergist for testing. But first try some of the following remedies for eradicating the environmental antagonists that sometimes trigger migraines and see if the changes make his headaches and other allergy symptoms less frequent.

- **Barrel into the bedroom:** Change bedding (sheets, blankets, mattress cover, bedspread) once a week, and replace pillowcases daily. Use hot water to wash bedding. Put coverings on mattresses and pillows to ward off the growth of mites in your bed dust. Don't let your child sleep on a feather pillow, because feathers can be allergens.

- **Make it easy to avoid triggers:** Help your child avoid plants, dust mites, mildew, animal dander, and insects such as cockroaches. Get him to help you in acclimating your indoor dog to being an outside dog.

- **Take household precautions:** Make sure that indoor appliances and fireplaces are well ventilated so that your child isn't subjected to carbon monoxide fumes. Ask smokers to go outside to smoke.

✔ **Keep a cleanliness checklist:** Keep the interiors of your home well dusted, mopped, and vacuumed to keep house dust to a minimum. Get rid of furniture and wall hangings that collect dust. Install air filtration devices for air purification. Frequently change air filters on air-conditioning and heating units.

✔ **Keep your child's stuff clean:** Frequently wash stuffed animals, pillows, and security blankets, because they can harbor allergens.

✔ **Do dust-mite busting:** Stave off dust mites with frequent cleanings of carpeting and rugs, and keep the humidity low and the temperature moderate (a balmy atmosphere helps dust mites thrive). Dust mites burrow in carpets and furniture and thrive in hot, wet rooms; they live off your ever-shedding skin cells and deposit waste pellets daily.

✔ **Protect your child:** Help him steer clear of pollen, fumes, mold, and allergens such as fresh-cut grass, fresh paint, hairspray, aerosol sprays, solvents, garbage odors, and cleaning chemicals.

Harnessing hormones

Puberty is by far the most common startup time for youngsters' migraines (although some kids are lucky enough to outgrow them eventually). And, throughout childhood, migraines often occur as sidekicks to common infections.

Boys have as many headaches as girls, if not more. But the gender gap widens permanently at the onset of adolescence. Menstrual hormones start rocking the boat, and girls begin to outnumber guys in the number and severity of headaches.

Many women begin to first have migraines during puberty, and some develop headaches only during their periods. Migraines can get worse (or better) during other times of shifting hormones: when you're taking birth control pills, when you're pregnant, or during the years of menopause, for example. For more on women's migraines, see Chapter 19.

At any rate, you can help your adolescent alleviate hormonal triggers by helping to implement the following suggestions:

✔ Avoid food triggers because they can join ranks with hormones and cause a migraine.

✔ Make lifestyle changes, such as stopping smoking, starting a walking program, and assessing the impact of birth-control pills on migraines.

✔ Take medications to help the pain and nausea/vomiting (see Chapters 7, 8, and 19 for information on helpful medications).

Replacing exercise that hurts with exercise that helps

Perhaps your child gets a migraine right after playing basketball or participating in gym class at school. Maybe your son's head starts to ache following football practice or a high-intensity karate class.

After your child has been evaluated by his healthcare provider and has been diagnosed with *exertional migraines* (and other problems have been ruled out), some possible remedies are

- Do a slow warm-up before beginning the activity.
- Take acetaminophen or ibuprofen before the physical exertion.
- Find a form of exercise (walking or cycling) that doesn't result in a migraine.
- Drink plenty of water to stay well hydrated before, during, and after exercising. (Dehydration can contribute to migraine development at any time.)

Resolving uneven sleep patterns

Uneven sleep patterns almost guarantee occasional head pain in children who have an inborn migraine tendency. What works much better with the ultra-sensitive systems of these young bodies is a structured sleep scene. If you make sure that the migraine-prone child has routine bedtimes and wake-up times, and the same number of hours of sleep per night, you'll be very likely to see a huge decrease in the number of headaches.

Here are ways to help shape up your youngster's sleep patterns:

- Avoid giving your child food or drinks that contain sugar or caffeine during the evening.
- Make sure your child is getting about 8 to 9 hours of sleep per night.
- See that your child goes to bed at about the same time every night, and wake him up at the same time each morning.

  If you follow this tip, your child will get approximately the same amount of sleep nightly. You can loosen up a bit on weekends, of course, when the whole family probably prefers to sleep a bit longer. But be careful here, because sleeping in can contribute to erratic sleep that may result in a migraine.

Dealing with stress and excitement

Kids get excited about upcoming trips, parties, and events. They sometimes dread tests and hate the prospect of speaking in front of a class at school. These are normal kinds of stress that come with growing up. But, like adults, kids may also face even greater stresses. Your child may feel responsible for your divorce and suffer super-sized stress due to his perception. Or he may dislike a certain teacher, caregiver, or bullying peer.

Of course, you can't take away life's bumps and detours, but you can help your migraine-prone child by showing him effective ways to deal with stress-and-joy triggers. As with adults, children may do really well using relaxation techniques and imagery (see Chapter 9).

You can also help your child reduce his stress by doing the following things:

- ✔ **Teach him to take breaks:** Encourage school-age kids to take homework and computer timeouts by getting up and moving around.

- ✔ **Give him a hug or massage:** Give your child frequent stress-relieving, reassuring hugs, or massage his upper back while he's at his desk studying.

- ✔ **Help him walk off anxiety:** Ask your child to join you on a walk, and encourage him to talk about things that are on his mind.

- ✔ **Prep him for new situations:** When he faces a change in routine (new school, new caregiver, field trip), role-play the experience ahead of time so that he gets psyched up for a good time rather than a scary one.

Seeking Treatment

Treating your child's head pain is often less difficult than defusing the ticking migraine bomb in a grownup's skull. Treatments for kids' migraines work! And, you have lots to choose from.

You can run the gamut, from home remedies to behavioral changes to prescription drugs, to find the solution for the migraine-plagued child in your life.

First try putting a cold pack on his hurting head and tucking him into bed in a dark room. If sleeping off the pain doesn't work, give him an over-the-counter medication. Follow the dosage recommendations on the bottle — proper doses depend on your child's weight, not age. If you're nervous about whether you're giving the right dose, check with your doctor's office for advice. If your child isn't experiencing nausea or vomiting with his headache, you can give him fruit juice or a snack if he's hungry.

Other treatments include magnesium supplements, prescription drugs, biofeedback, imagery, and relaxation techniques.

Trying home remedies

Before you decide how to treat your child's migraines, consider the age of the youngster and the frequency/severity of his headaches. A very young child (five or younger) may benefit from taking a mild over-the-counter (OTC) medicine and spending an hour sleeping off the pain, whereas an older child may need a more aggressive headache treatment.

When giving OTC medications, follow dose recommendations on the bottle. If you feel shaky about giving your child a medication, it's fine to check with your doctor's office to confirm that you're doing the right thing. (When in doubt, check it out.)

Don't give aspirin to a child younger than 14 years old. Reye's syndrome, a serious neurological disorder, has been linked to aspirin use in children. Good alternatives are the pain relievers ibuprofen and acetaminophen. (You can check labels to make sure that pain relievers don't have aspirin.)

If you give your child OTC pain medication, and his headache persists for more than 24 hours, call your doctor.

Home remedies can be good first approaches for children five and older, too, but if the simple stuff fails to work, try having your child avoid known migraine triggers and use relaxation techniques, imagery, or biofeedback. (See Chapter 9 for info on these and other alternative treatments.) If necessary, move from home remedies up to the next level of migraine-busting — prescription medications.

If you and your child have trouble pinpointing his food triggers, you may want to try an elimination diet, which can usually unmask troublemakers at the dinner table. (See the elimination diet in Chapter 11.) The elimination diet should be a last-resort measure, though, because it's especially tough for kids to follow strict dietary rules.

If the simple measures don't help, take your child to see a pediatrician or family practice doctor for treatment.

You may be able to manage your child's migraines with one of the following home treatments:

✔ Give your child ibuprofen, acetaminophen, or naproxen at the onset of his headache, and have him lie down to rest or sleep. (Follow your doctor's advice or the package's instructions for dosing appropriate to your child's weight and age.)

If he continues to feel bad, you can repeat the dosing as recommended on the label. (If you have questions, check with your child's doctor.)

✔ Try giving your child a caffeinated soft drink — the caffeine may help eliminate the pain, and it can also make pills go down more easily. Caffeine can be a migraine trigger for some children, but it may also work as a headache pain reliever. If you know that caffeine is a headache trigger for your child, substitute a glass of water.

✔ Show your child how to experiment with relaxation techniques. Your child may get pain relief from biofeedback or deep breathing. (See Chapter 9 for more on these techniques.)

Kids are excellent at using imagery. Tell your child to imagine that he can see the blood pumping through his blood vessels, working its way down to warm the chilly hands and feet that are often migraine symptoms. Tell him that he can create this picture in his mind any time he wants to. For many children, this technique helps relieve pain.

Children are likely to be nauseated with a migraine, so keep a basin nearby. See Figure 20-1.

Your child may get enthusiastic about looking for ways to handle his migraines and find his triggers. Because these headaches are highly individual in nature, the sooner a youngster learns to manage the headaches himself, the better off he'll be.

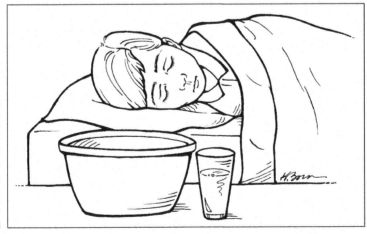

Figure 20-1:
Keeping a basin near a migraine-stricken child is a good idea.

Going to the doctor

Don't fool around with childhood headaches. If your child doesn't get relief from the pain and other symptoms after 24 hours of home remedies, see your healthcare provider so that the three of you can work up a plan for the migraine dilemma. You may want to take a headache journal with you (see the headache journal in Chapter 3.)

Get in the habit of being an advocate for your child's health (and your own). Of course, most doctors try to be extremely thorough and careful, but it never hurts to underscore a special health condition that may have gone unnoticed on your tot's medical chart.

Getting a diagnosis

When a child does have migraines, getting them diagnosed is important. In the doctor's office, the physical exam may include

- ✔ **Measuring head circumference:** Your child's doctor checks for normal development of the skull. An excessive head-growth rate can point to increased intracranial pressure, which may be caused by tumors or *hydrocephalus* (an enlargement of ventricles in the brain due to an abnormal increase in cerebrospinal fluid.)

- ✔ **Blood pressure and temperature check:** The doctor checks your child's temperature to make sure that your child doesn't have fever, which can indicate an infection.

- ✔ **Tooth inspection:** The doctor checks for cavities or a tooth abscess that may be causing your child's headaches.

- ✔ **Examination for signs of sinusitis:** Your doctor wants to determine if your child has sinusitis, because the condition can cause headaches.

- ✔ **Neurological exam:** This part of the physical checks out the status of your child's cranial nerves, reflexes, coordination, and so on.

Typically, your doctor will want some information about your child's head-pain episodes. The doctor will also ask you and your child questions to help determine what kind of headaches your child has:

- ✔ **Onset and frequency:** How often does he have headaches and how long has he been having them? What time of day do his headaches usually occur? Have his headaches increased in number or severity? How long do his headaches last?

- ✔ **Headache characteristics:** How does he describe the pain, and where does it hurt — one side of his head or both? Are there other symptoms before, during, or after his headaches — weakness, tiredness, nausea, vomiting, or visual disturbances? Does he ever have unexplained vomiting/nausea without a headache?

✔ **Headache causes and triggers:** Have you noticed anything that seems to make his headaches worse (noise, bright lights, exercise, coughing, stressors at school or home, lack of sleep, certain foods)? Has your child fallen and hit his head recently? Is there a family history of headaches? Do you have migraines? Does another family member have them?

✔ **Headache treatments:** What helps him get over a headache (sleep, cold cloth on his head, quiet)? What kinds of medications have you tried, and did they help?

✔ **Odds and ends:** Does he have motion sickness? Was he a colicky infant?

In rare cases, the doctor may order some tests. He may want to do a CT (computerized tomography) scan, or CAT scan, of the head to check for a tumor or other abnormality. Or he may want to do an MRI (magnetic resonance imaging) of the brain to look for *vascular* (blood vessel) abnormalities. In some cases, a lumbar puncture, or spinal tap, may be necessary to evaluate for possible meningitis. (See Chapter 6 for more information on tests.) Alternatively, your doctor may want you to take your child to see a specialist, such as a neurologist.

If answers to your child's headache are hard to find, the doctor may also evaluate your child for some other, very rare, headache syndromes.

Filling a prescription

Your doctor likely will prescribe medication if the remedies you've tried don't help your child's pain and nausea.

If your doctor prescribes medication, ask what side effects you can expect. Make sure that you understand the amount of medicine to give your child and the frequency with which you should give it. In addition, ask questions such as, "So, can I presume that this medication is safe even though Nicholas has asthma?" You definitely want to ask if the drug will be safe for your child if he has existing medical problems.

If your kid is a picky pill-taker, ask your doctor if the medication also comes in a flavored liquid version.

Abortive medications (drugs that help stop an existing headache) can often provide migraine pain relief for children. For the possible side effects associated with these drugs, see Chapter 8.

The abortives include the following drugs:

✔ **Non-steroidal anti-inflammatory drugs:** A prescription form of naproxen is available.

✔ **Midrin:** This drug is referred to as a *combination medication* because it's a combo of several medicines, and it doesn't belong in any of the other groupings of migraine drugs.

- ✔ **The triptans:** Imitrex (nasal spray and pill form), Maxalt, and Amerge are all triptans, which are a highly effective group of migraine medications that have revolutionized migraine treatment because of their effectiveness. These are not FDA-approved for use in children, but physicians do prescribe them, and studies are under way.

- ✔ **Intravenous DHE (dihydroergotamine mesylate):** This drug is delivered into the vein by needle and used in the case of very severe migraine attacks. Metoclopramide (for nausea and vomiting) is given orally or intravenously before the DHE.

If your child has disabling migraines that result in significant problems with inactivity and school absences, preventives (medications used to prevent migraines) may be prescribed for him to take on a daily basis for a set period of time. (See Chapter 8 for more on preventatives.) After that period, you meet with your doctor for a reassessment of the migraines to decide if your child should continue taking the medication.

Preventives include the following:

- ✔ **Cyproheptadine (Periactin):** This drug is chiefly used in young children ages 2 to 12.

- ✔ **Nonsteroidal anti-inflammatory drugs:** Used to relieve pain and reduce swelling, these drugs include naproxene, ketoprofen, and beta blockers. (The beta blocker propranolol shouldn't be used in patients with asthma, diabetes, and other special conditions).

- ✔ **Calcium channel blockers:** verapamil and diltiazem.

- ✔ **Anti-convulsants:** This sounds scarier than it is. Anticonvulsants are just a class of medication that's been found to relieve migraines. Although it hasn't been well studied in children, Depakote may be used to treat migraines.

- ✔ **Tricyclic antidepressants:** Amitriptyline (Elavil) is one of a major class of medications that work for migraines. *Tricyclic* refers to the structure of molecule — we know, more information than you needed.

Doctors often prescribe Phenergan (promethazine) to treat the nausea and vomiting of migraines. The medication can be given orally or rectally. Other drugs used to relieve nausea and/or vomiting are metoclopramide and chlorpromazine.

Phenergan is often given by *rectal suppository* (a capsule that you insert into the child's anus). You can expect your child to dislike this solution, so be sympathetic. At the same time, be matter-of-fact, letting him know that you both need to do whatever it takes to reach the goal of making him feel better and getting him back to enjoying life.

Have an adult (you or another caregiver) act as dispenser of medication for children who are 12 or younger. For kids older than 12, monitor drug use carefully and often.

Never give your child someone else's prescription drug. When you're dealing with children, their size, age, and other medical conditions determine dosing. You don't want to overmedicate.

Managing the Emotional Side Effects

You want your child to flourish. You hope to raise a strong, capable, happy youngster who faces challenges with confidence and aplomb. And, somehow, seeing him curled up on the bed in the fetal position, crying from the pain of an awful headache, just doesn't fit.

But you can definitely take charge of the situation. Be the one who transitions your child seamlessly from headache days to healthy days. Show him how to finesse the problem. Exude optimism and can-do spirit: These enormous assets can be contagious. (As a matter of fact, you may have a good background for helping your migraine kid if you're a migraine sufferer yourself.)

Be honest and upfront. Let your child know that you feel conflict when helping him through his migraine because you truly regard headache pain as genuinely awful, but you also want him to develop a good work ethic. Thinking of headache days as fallback positions isn't good, because he may begin to look at himself as being disabled. Many migraineurs find out that they can sometimes shake the pain if they get out of the house and do things rather than give in and retreat to bed. On the other hand, going to bed after taking a migraine medication is not at all unusual for some people. Oftentimes, it's the only way to go.

Headaches that are bad enough to make a child unable to cope with school or other activities affect about one out of ten kids in the 10 to 19 age bracket. Being sidelined by migraines is no small issue.

Addressing the lame-headache-kid image

A low self-image is often a big problem for children who suffer from migraines. Don't be surprised if your child turns to you with the "Why me?" question. Coming up with an answer can be quite a quandary, all right. Nevertheless, developing a habit of positive thinking is a good coping tool for any hurdle your child may encounter.

Remembering that children will key into an adult's response to the migraine is important. Recall the times when your child fell down and scraped his knee; if he looked at you and you were upset, he got upset. If you were matter-of-fact — got him up and back into action quickly — he didn't look at the injury as a crisis. He rallied in no time.

Often, your child may feel somewhat out-of-step or disadvantaged by missing activities and school due to migraines — a situation that can lead to a diminished sense of self. The following tips can help you address this problem:

- **Play up his strengths.** Any child with a chronic illness needs to be led to focus on all the good qualities he has. Tell him: "No one gets through life without aches and pains, but who has the kind of sense of humor you do?" Or "Who can draw like you can?" Or "Who is so well liked by friends?"

- **Model a positive approach if you're also a migraine sufferer.** Your child will be watching to see if you get yourself moving on headache days or if you fall back under the covers. (Hypochondriacs aren't born. They're molded and fussed over — in many cases — by overly indulgent but well-meaning parents.)

- **Cite examples of pop-culture icons who have migraines.** You can name pro athletes, singers, musicians, or actors. This information can help make your child feel less alone and more like he's in good company. Elvis was a migraineur. Model Elle Macpherson has had her share of migraine pain, and so has basketball superstar Steve Francis of the Houston Rockets. ("Hey, kid! You rock, just like some other folks with migraines!")

- **Make sure that you tell him that he doesn't get migraine attacks because he's been bad.** Some young children may think that the Great Big Goblin Headache-Giver in the Sky is punishing their occasional naughtiness.

You can easily turn a migraine-suffering kid into a semi-invalid when he's sick. Sure, you're dying to comfort your child. However, the kid who's encouraged to get up and get out develops a can-do attitude, which is always an asset. On the other hand, if you teach him to avoid handling adversity, and you're always nursing his "war wounds," it's all too easy for the migraine child to become a social outcast who's isolated from his peers and sees himself as fragile and disadvantaged.

Deciding whether to send him to school with a headache

Many children rate just being at school as a major headache trigger. For the headache-prone, the whirlwind atmosphere of school — with its noise, bright lights, and peer troubles (bullying and harassment) — can result in severe and frequent migraines.

What's a parent to do? Part of you wants to send your child to school when he has a headache, so he won't get a reputation for being a slacker non-attendee wimp. However, you also know that if he does go, he'll be in for a rough day of trying to cope with peers, lessons, and teachers while a concrete drill is rat-tat-tatting in his head. Also, his self-image may suffer if he performs poorly, which is likely to be the case when head pain makes it hard to concentrate.

On the other hand, if you don't send your child to school, he can get stressed from missing classes, and he may wind up feeling like a misfit. Getting behind in studies, sports, and social activities can be a real disappointment for a kid.

Is this a time to push a little, or a time to be a buffer, asking for your child to be excused from school? Or should you just get him a doctor's note to get out of participating in gym or track?

We offer these tips for handling school issues for your migraine-suffering child:

✔ **Weigh the risk/benefit columns of attendance versus non-attendance on migraine days.** At a time when he's pain-free, get your child to sit down and help you list the pros and cons of going to school with a headache. Pros of attending would be that he doesn't get behind, he gets to see his friends, and he feels like he knows what's going on. Cons of going to school when hampered by head pain are the glazed-mind spin-offs: seeming unresponsive to teachers and friends, failing to do good work, or making people mad because he feels bad and moody.

You may think that you're oh-so-clued-in to what bothers your child the most about missing school or what's troublesome about going to school with a headache, but you may not necessarily be right on target. Let him talk; you may be surprised at what you hear. Don't forget, it's his head and his life.

✔ **Consult with your doctor to come up with a headache management strategy that you can share with the school.** If your child needs medication on occasion, the school nurse needs information on file about the required doses. The school will also need to know if your child requires an hour or so to lie down in the school clinic from time to time.

✔ **Come up with a school-versus-no-school game plan for migraine days.** If you come up with a game plan, you won't have to deal with this issue time after time and keep feeling anxious over what may be the better approach.

✔ **Encourage your child to go to school if the pain is just "nagging."** Tell your child to let you know when he's too miserable to be in a learning frame of mind. Sometimes, going to bed to sleep off a headache is absolutely the best (and only) thing to do.

I am so not worthy. *Hello!* I am worthy!

For many people, the roots of migraine management begin in the formative years. One adult migraineur (Calvin, now 55) recalls that when his migraines were diagnosed at age 5, his mother seemed angry with him. She gave him an aspirin, put him to bed in a dark room, and treated him like an invalid. As one of seven children, Calvin never got his mother's undivided attention except during headache episodes — but he still got the impression that she liked his brothers, who were "less trouble" because they weren't migraine-sufferers, better. So, for Calvin, migraines became an agony/ecstasy thing. These migraines were legitimate biological pain-causers, all right, but they were also sad forms of getting attention.

When he became an adult, still suffering incapacitating frequent migraines, he routinely called in sick; he would pop a pain pill and sleep off the pain. Taught early in life that he was "handicapped," Calvin made no attempt to work through the headaches until he read an article that described an alternate approach. At age 39, he discovered that he could take his medication and go to work; to his surprise, being active helped him get rid of headaches more quickly than sleeping did. In addition, he reduced his amount of unproductive time, which had always been unsettling to him. So, in middle age, he reframed his idea of what migraines meant and followed a new battle anthem.

The moral of the story: The wise and compassionate handling of a migraine kid can massively mold his lifelong self-image. As any motivational speaker will tell you, "You are what you think you are." Perception is everything.

So, if you give your migraine child the poor-pitiful-me crutch, he may pick it up and wield it as a good excuse for not trying. But if you tell him he's wonderful, capable, and one-of-a-kind — hey, everyone has a few aches and pains — he'll embrace the I-am-worthy platform. Think how cool that will be.

Give your child lots of praise when he toughs it out on headache days. If he manages to take part in a class or activity, he definitely deserves congratulations and a pat on the back.

Let your child know (gently) that someday, in adulthood, he'll face days when he's not feeling up to par but really must show up and cope with his workday, nonetheless. (See the sidebar titled "I am so not worthy. *Hello!* I am worthy!")

Chapter 21

Holding Off the Sex Migraine

. . . .

In This Chapter

▶ Feeling the confusion of a sex-headache blast

▶ Having a frank talk with your doctor

▶ Treating sex migraines appropriately so you don't have to skip having sex

. . . .

*E*ver hear of an orgasmic thunderclap? This type of headache, which is also referred to as a sex headache, is a very nasty offshoot of your sexuality.

The fact is, any kind of exertion, including exercise, can make a migraine blossom or worsen. It just so happens that sex can sometimes be a fairly rambunctious undertaking. Experts think that the exertion factor is why sexual activity can trigger a severe and sudden migraine in some people — mostly men.

Most sexual headaches are obnoxious but harmless. They should be given a careful look and evaluation, though, because they aren't always benign. In fact, sexual headaches sometimes occur because of a *hemorrhage* (bleeding) in the brain.

If you experience a first-ever or worst-ever headache during or after sex, you definitely need to seek evaluation to rule out the possibility of a very serious health condition. If you experience recurrent headaches with sex, you also need to be evaluated by a healthcare provider.

This chapter fills you in on the common symptoms of orgasmic headaches. It also covers the medications you can use to get headache relief and resume a normal sex life.

Laying Out Sex-Related Headaches

Three types of benign headaches are associated with sex:

- ✔ A dull head pain that appears to result from head-and-neck muscle contractions during the arousal/excitement of sexual activity.

- ✔ An intense headache called an orgasmic migraine, or orgasmic cephalalgia, which usually features generalized head pain that hits like a bolt from out of nowhere at the time of orgasm (This is the most common type of sex headache).

- ✔ A headache that occurs after sex with a change in posture. (Any move, such as rolling apart or standing up, can kick off this often excruciating pain.)

If you have a thunderbolt headache during sex, and you've never experienced this type of headache previously during sex, see a doctor as soon as possible! Other accompanying signs that make a trip to the ER an absolute-must include any sort of neck rigidity with the headache, vomiting, irregular breathing, problems with coordination, and unresponsiveness. Even though most sex migraines don't require treatment, be sure to have the situation evaluated (just to take good care of yourself).

As Houston neurologist Brian Loftus explains, "There is nothing in history about a headache at the onset of orgasm (when blood pressure rises) that allows you to know it is not a subarachnoid bleed [bleeding in the brain]. Even if a person's exam is normal when I see him, I have to consider a warning bleed. Now if someone comes to me with a 20-year history of headaches during sex and exertion that he has had on multiple occasions each year, then of course I would not bother with any scan or tap (assuming the patient's neurological exam is normal), as no one has 100 warning bleeds without the big one."

Sex headaches aren't always innocent

One doctor tells of a young woman who had sex headaches and was first told that she had a benign condition. It was later discovered that she had two aneurysms, one of which had ruptured to produce a subarachnoid hemorrhage — a potentially life-threatening condition. In her case, both aneurysms were surgically clipped, saving her life.

Anyone who has a so-called benign sex headache should go to a doctor for evaluation initially to exclude the possibility of a very serious health condition.

Headaches that occur with orgasm can be a symptom of a stroke, a tumor, or bleeding in your brain (a brain hemorrhage), so it's important to get them checked out the first time they occur.

You don't have to have a partner for sex-related headaches to hit. Solo sex activity can bring them on, too.

So what's a sex headache all about? Here are some of the characteristics of sex migraines:

- **The bombshell look:** You may look (and feel) as though you've been hit by a missile. Shocked by the sudden pain, you may grab your head and whimper or moan.

- **Very bad timing:** To make matters worse, the explosive type of head pain usually devastates you just at the moment you experience orgasm.

- **Short but not sweet:** These headaches are short-lived. Often, they subside a few minutes after orgasm. Occasionally, they may last for hours.

- **Slow creeper:** For some folks, sex headaches start with a dull roar during sexual activity and unload their real blast of pain at the time of orgasm.

- **Likes men better:** For some unknown reason, men have sex headaches much more often than women do.

If a sudden-onset headache happens to you — either during or right at the time of orgasm — the first thing you need to do is forget about sex immediately. No more sex for the time being! Stopping sex will probably eliminate the pain; you may feel it diminish quickly as your body calms down and gets back to normal pacing.

Researchers and physicians conjecture that sex headaches are caused when exertion greatly increases blood flow and dilates blood vessels — a common trigger for migraines.

You won't know for sure if a thunderclap headache signals that your health is in jeopardy. If you've experienced sex headaches in the past, and you've felt them fade away right after orgasm, the chances are good that they'll fade the next time, too. But be alert for any signs that make your headaches different or worse. If you have a headache that doesn't go away after a couple of minutes or hours like the previous one(s), for example, see a doctor to have it checked out.

Having a Candid Chat with Your Doctor

To find something that works for a sex migraine, you may need to try several different medications over a period of time. The more information you provide your doctor, the better she can prescribe the right drug. So don't be afraid to be perfectly honest with your doctor.

Your doctor can look at your headache history to see if there's an obvious cause for the trouble you're having. If she's not able to determine the cause from your medical history, she'll dig further and find out what's going on.

If you persevere with fact-finding, it's very likely that you and your doctor will find an answer to your problem.

Giving a doctor sketchy, incomplete information on a health problem related to sex is the norm rather than the exception. So try your best to leapfrog over your reticence about discussing personal matters, and tell your doctor all the pertinent information that she may be able to use to diagnose what's wrong. She's not going to judge your sex life. It's her job to help you solve your problem.

You need to be forthcoming about your sex headaches for two main reasons:

- ✔ You may have a life-threatening condition that requires testing and treatment.

- ✔ You need to find a solution for your headaches, because sex-related problems often make people steer clear of sexual activity, and having a sexual release is important to your overall health.

Just because you have a history of migraines doesn't rule out the possibility that you may be stricken with a headache that is indicative of a life-threatening condition. If in doubt, see your doctor to have your condition checked out.

Doing It without Getting Done In

Perhaps you really don't want to join an order of people who take celibacy vows. Fact is, if you wanted to become a nun or a monk, you probably would have decided this before you started engaging in sexual activity, right?

So your goal in the headache arena is to find a way that you can still have sex but not face the horrible headaches that can come in tandem with orgasm. These headaches are a no-fun aspect of sex and can be enough to make almost anyone shy away from repeat sexual encounters.

After a doctor has evaluated you, performed any necessary tests, and determined that you're having benign sex headaches, your options are

- ✔ Over-the-counter pain relief for sex headaches that persist

- ✔ A prescription medication if mild pain killers don't help

- ✔ A prescription medication that you take before having sex to try to ward off an explosive headache

Trying over-the-counter analgesics

You may want to try taking an over-the-counter (OTC) pain pill before you participate in any kind of sexual activity.

The drug of choice is usually a nonsteroidal anti-inflammatory such as naproxen (Aleve). Take the recommended dose prior to starting any kind of sexual activity, whether with a partner or solo.

Getting a prescription medication

If you keep having sex headaches, your doctor may decide to prescribe a preventive drug, such as indomethacin (Indocin) or the beta blocker propranolol (Inderal), so that you can ward off repeat headaches. Or she may prescribe a medication to take as needed for the pain of a sex headache. You usually take preventive medicine on a regular basis only in special instances (see Chapter 8 for reasons that people use prophylactic migraine medications).

Don't be afraid to use your usual prescription migraine drug for sexual headaches. But take the medication exactly the way your doctor recommends. Don't use more pills than you're supposed to, and don't use them more frequently than you're supposed to.

Chances are good that any headaches that come galloping along with your sexual climax can simply be labeled "benign sexual headaches." You treat them with medication before or after sex, and you deal with the problem effectively.

Getting help for sex-related anxiety

If you often experience sex headaches when you have an orgasm, your interest in having sex may drop dramatically. If pleasure has to be associated with that kind of pain, who needs it, right?

Taking care of your partner

"I'm so worried about my husband because his head almost explodes after orgasm. This used to happen now and then, but it has become the norm. I've tried to get him to see a doctor, but he refuses because the headache goes away so quickly. So I asked my gynecologist if this could be a sign of something serious."

This woman's doctor suggested that she should persuade her husband to see a doctor for evaluation. Although he said it was probably just benign sex headaches, the fact that they were becoming more frequent was good enough reason to get him checked out.

When she told her husband that worsening severe headaches were sometimes symptomatic of serious conditions such as a brain tumor or hemorrhage, he was willing to see a doctor. The internist who evaluated the man ordered a CT scan, which came up normal. He then performed a *lumbar puncture* (spinal tap), which also showed normal. These tests essentially ruled out anything other than what is usually the case when someone has a bad headache during or after orgasm — a benign sex headache. The doctor recommended that they try sexual abstinence for a couple of weeks to see if it would help, and then if the problem continued, he should take a nonsteroidal anti-inflammatory, such as Aleve, an hour before sex to prevent the onset of a headache.

The doctor explained to the couple that while sex headaches are clearly irritants, they're usually harmless, and only a small percentage are caused by a serious condition. But that offhand possibility of a life-threatening condition makes emergency medical evaluation important for someone who's experiencing a new-onset headache during sex.

If you face this predicament, try using relaxation techniques. They may help reduce the anxiety that stems from the fear that you'll get a migraine every time you have sex. (See Chapter 9 for more on relaxation techniques.)

You don't want to skip sex entirely, because the physical release of orgasm is important to your overall health and sense of well-being.

Chapter 22

Sideswiping Migraines Caused by Stress

. . . .

In This Chapter

▶ Mastering mind-calming techniques

▶ Eliminating stressors

. . . .

Divorce and child support. Disintegrating families and violence. Information overload and technology overkill. Global disasters and terrorists. We all face a multitude of existing (and imagined) threats and problems. So you obsess a bit. And if you have a migraine tendency, you're likely to find all of your stressors ganging up with your headache triggers to produce head pain.

Stress can crop up anywhere: work, home, freeways, malls, grocery stores, or church. Undeniably, you'll never manage to eliminate all stressors from your lifestyle. So it's best to accept that you're going to face plenty of them and go to work on tempering the impact that stress can have on your life. Even if you could make your life completely stress-free, it wouldn't necessarily be a good thing. Stress can be a positive in that it nudges you to action, helps you take on challenges, and allows you to move forward. But it can also be guilty of teaming up with other migraine triggers and wreaking havoc in your brain.

You can combat stress with relaxation techniques and biofeedback (see Chapter 9), and behavior modification (see the following section). Mind-calming techniques, such as self-talk and reframing, can be used to make your body less likely to crank up stress levels that may lead to migraines.

Because it seems clear that stress can antagonize your brain's sensitive neurons, the sooner you figure out how to avoid meltdowns, the less often you'll see stress joining ranks with other trigger punks and causing a migraine.

Mastering Techniques for Calming Your Mind

As an aggravator of headaches, a stress spiral works like this: The hormones adrenaline and cortisol go into overdrive when you're stressed, pumping up your heart rate and blood pressure, which may lead to blood-vessel changes that result in headache pain.

Aside from whatever else is going on in your head, your mind can be extremely powerful in moderating how stress affects you in your daily life — your perception of events and your ways of coping with them. Most doctors believe that, to some degree, you can think yourself sick — or well.

The key skill you need in your coping backpack is a way (or ways) to make sure that stress doesn't disable you. When you arm yourself with a few techniques that fit your personality, you can handle stress in a way that makes you less anxious and more proactive. If you can fret less, stress will be less likely to do a job on your head.

You can become an expert at self-talking your way down from high-wire stress. And you can practice reframing events so that things that used to seem overwhelming become events that you can take in stride. As the islanders say, "No problem, mon."

Choosing positive approaches

You can choose to give tough situations a positive tilt. To do this, though, you may have to abandon your habit of being a worrywart who obsesses about "what if this happens?" and "what if that happens?"

Certainly one of the most effective ways to quit worrying is to ask yourself, "What's the worst thing that can happen if my fears do come true?" You look at the worst possible outcome; acknowledge that while it may be unfortunate, it's probably not terminal; and get on with your day.

Getting with the game plan

You can examine any problem and list several ways to solve it instead of let yourself get carried away with doomsday-scenario thinking.

Perhaps you fear getting dumped by your mate. Your marriage isn't going well, and you're pretty sure that you'll be getting a pink slip from her very soon.

You can handle this problem by setting up a game plan for what you can do. Instead of spending so much time borrowing trouble, just presume that the worst is going to happen and draw up a one-two-three plan of action. With this type of plan, you discover that you have options:

- ✔ See a therapist for counseling to get you through your distress.

- ✔ Take up a new hobby as a distraction to keep you from jumping on the dating bandwagon too soon. (Heal for at least six months before dating.)

- ✔ Do as Dr. Phil (of Oprah fame) suggests — perform an "autopsy" on your dead relationship and try to learn something from what went wrong.

- ✔ List your good qualities and play them up. Pat yourself on the back and remind yourself that some people you know really appreciate these qualities.

- ✔ List the qualities you want to work on.

- ✔ Check to see what happened to you as a result of the split (Did you die? Did you go crazy?). If you didn't self-destruct, you're probably going to be all right.

Reframing a problem

The problem: You don't have enough money (the same head-scratcher that lots of people struggle with). You can't quite cover your bills, and you certainly don't have enough to sock away savings. The cause: Your profession is low-paying. You enjoy what you do, but you don't enjoy being strapped financially.

You can start a stress-worry cycle, thinking "I don't know what I'm going to do! There's no answer to this!" Or you can reframe the problem: Instead of concluding that your financial picture is impossible and stewing in worry and despair, you're going to lay out some possible solutions. Following are some options you may consider:

- ✔ Borrow money for the things you want.

- ✔ Find another job that's not as much fun but pays more.

- ✔ Find a job you like that pays more.

- ✔ Look for supplemental income sources — consulting work, or freelance or contract opportunities.

Now dissect the options and choose the one you can deal with most easily. Suddenly what looked like a dismal dilemma has been reframed into a more favorable and flattering light and made doable. You can reevaluate your choice at any time.

Adjusting your attitude about migraines

You can easily let yourself feel demoralized and discouraged because your life isn't pain-free and no one understands how much you hurt at times, or you can reframe your situation in the following ways:

✔ **Accept what is.** Although it may not feel fair that you have to put up with headaches, there are plenty of people with much worse health maladies. So count your blessings and practice acceptance.

✔ **Decide what you want to do in your life.** Set up goals and decide how you're going to get there. You lower your stress by feeling empowered and in charge rather than feeling as though you're a victim of the whims of fate.

✔ **Define yourself as an upbeat, involved, can-do individual.** Don't let anyone or any number of headaches tell you any different. Vow not to think of yourself as disabled and understand clearly that how you name your problem (migraines) helps determine the role it plays in your life.

✔ **Be proactive.** Do the smart things that help you manage your headaches well: proper exercise (see Chapter 12), avoidance of food triggers (Chapter 11), proper rest (see Chapter 14), use of relaxation techniques (Chapter 9), and the use (but not overuse) of migraine medications (see Chapters 7 and 8).

✔ **Show healthy behaviors at home and work.** Don't expect the world to revolve around your headache tendency — roll with the punches and make your own way. Remember that millions of people have health problems that they have to live with and work around.

✔ **Get good at applying your coping strategies.** Handle stress in a way that keeps it from being a major factor in your development of migraines. Stress is one of many possible migraine triggers, so you should discover how to put a lid on the habit of needless worry.

Using self-talk to prevent big, bad migraines

You can use the self-talk method of reducing stress to make anxiety and stress less likely to gang up with other migraine-trigger bums and haunt your brain.

If you're like most people, you may have a tendency to tell yourself that you're not good at doing certain things. But you need to get into the habit of taking the opposite approach. Tell yourself that you're going to knock 'em dead and be well prepared, and you'll likely be successful in the endeavors you undertake.

Positive self-talk may ratchet down the severity of a migraine or help keep one from developing. You can also use it as a stress-reduction tool that can make migraines less apt to happen.

Be sure to use messages that psych you up for the expectation of doing well. For example, you may want to use the following type of mental self-talk before giving an important sales presentation for your company: "People are going to be wowed by how prepared I am. I expect to find these clients very interested in doing business by the time I get through. I will be articulate. I will smile and act relaxed. I will ask for their feedback and show that I care about understanding their business needs."

Okay, now that you have the gist of the process, try using self-talk to ratchet up your ability to handle stress and experience less anxiety. Hopefully you can convert your stress into the walking wounded rather than an able soldier in stirring up migraine action.

Rearranging Priorities to Scuttle Some Stressors

Feeling aimless, disorganized, or scattered can contribute to your Stress Crucible. You can improve your situation by discovering how to rearrange your priorities. When you rearrange your priorities, you automatically scuttle the stressors that come with not having your act together.

You can steer clear of people and things that tend to increase your stress level. Why put yourself in the position of feeling anxious if you don't have to?

Be logical and smart. Take care of yourself, and get yourself into a stress-scuttling frame of mind.

Organizing stress-free days

If you're basically an unstructured person (sometimes known as a mess), how do you get organized? Some people say that it's impossible to change your erratic ways, but it's actually one of the easiest things to change.

To become more organized, try doing the following:

- ✔ Evaluate your systems at home and work to decide whether they're working for you. Decide on a place for everything — and keep things in their places.

  Keeping things where you'll first think to look for them is a simple and effective organizing philosophy.

- ✔ Have a plan for your day and week. You can use a planner, a Palm Pilot, or a simple checklist.

  - Start each day by reviewing your day's plan.

  - Designate which tasks should be done first (very important), second (somewhat important), and last (not important).

- If possible, take care of your top priorities in the morning, when your energy level is high and your mind is fresh. That way, if you get off track because of emergencies or distractions, you'll have managed to cross off the most important items on your list.

- Put a few easy (or already-finished) tasks on your list so that you can cross them off and get into a groove. ("Hey, this feels good — I can do this!")

Avoiding the people and situations that stress you out

You may find yourself butting heads with situations and people who always cause you high stress. Why do you do this to yourself?

Instead, figure out if you really need to be around those folks who contribute to your stress. And if there are specific things or activities that make you feel anxious, do you really have to do them — or submit yourself to them?

You can handle these stressful situations with the following tips:

- ✔ **Set up defined times to deal with problem people or situations.** You have a dreaded meeting with your child's third-grade teacher. This wacky guy drives you nuts because he rattles on endlessly. You can't avoid him entirely, but you can set up meetings with specific ending times (you have an appointment, you must make a call, and so on). Take control.

- ✔ **Tweak standoffs your own way.** You may hate pressure-cooker situations with your stress-evoking boss, but there is something you can do to make them less stressful — bend these encounters to your advantage. Go into these meetings with a list of your own questions and a readiness to take notes. Be polite and efficient, and avoid small talk. This approach is not only professional, but it gets you in and out of there fast. Less muss and fuss. Less stress.

- ✔ **Prepare for stressors.** Get a handle on managing stressful situations that are unavoidable. For example, if you know that you have to spend holidays at your in-laws' home, and they always bicker and gossip to the point that it drives you up the wall, limit your exposure. Make a list of things to talk about (positive subjects!), and don't feel as though you have to submit to their bummer topics the whole time you're there. Seek out and pal around with the family member you like best.

- ✔ **Try an all-new tack.** Making even small changes in your own perspective can sometimes yield large rewards. For example, if your child whines and cries while you cook dinner, and nothing you can say seems to help, do something different. Get down on his level, look him in the eye, and ask if he wants to help. Give him a tiny task; make him feel valued and loved. Turn dinner preparation into a family enterprise, and you may shed stress in the process.

One of life's true ironies is that we worry ourselves silly about the opinions of people we don't even really like. Consider your hand-wringing, nail-biting feelings when you visit these thought processes: "What does he think of me?" "What can I do about that?" "He's always saying horrible things about people, so I know I'll be on his list at some point."

Try to release yourself from the grip of living in others' opinions. Absolutely *do* care what loved ones (friends and relatives) think about you, and try to make them proud with exemplary behaviors. But *don't* care what strangers and adversaries think of you. These people have very little to do with your life — this should clue you into how very little time you should spend worrying about what they think of you. They probably don't know you, and perhaps they don't want to. And that's okay. You don't have to please the world.

Find ways to loosen the stress vise that's hampering your quality of life and contributing to the evolution of migraines.

Getting his ducks in a row

A swinging single guy we know just couldn't seem to get organized. His haphazard ways were actually jeopardizing his job. This situation led to stress, which contributed to his developing migraines — or at least, that was his assessment of the chain of events.

He got anxious. He worried that his boss would find out that he wasn't up to speed for a big meeting. Soon, his head started pounding, making him even less capable of pulling off a professional presentation. And, not surprisingly, he bombed in a few meetings.

Finally, this guy decided to come up with some rules for his out-of-control lifestyle: Stop all of the late-night clubbing during the week; work on

organizational skills; spend time each morning prioritizing duties for the day; and take migraine medication as soon as a headache starts.

"I figured things couldn't be much worse," he said candidly. "I had nowhere to go but up."

After a month of being strict with himself, he made strides in improving his work ethic and performance. He's still no Gordon Gekko, top-achieving model of organization, but he's doing much better.

"And I don't feel so anxious all the time," he adds. "I feel like my stress migraine trigger won't detonate again very easily. I'm not freaking out over fear of losing my job anymore."

Chapter 23

The Senioring Effect: Aging and Migraines

. . . .

In This Chapter

▶ Getting fewer migraines (some seniors' lucky fate!)

▶ Experiencing migraines for the first time ever

▶ Meeting with your doctor to get answers and treat your problem

▶ Being on the lookout for eye problems and abnormal head pain

. . . .

*J*ust when you begin to wonder if there really are any advantages to getting older (other than senior discounts), someone tells you the good news about migraines. Many migraine sufferers who have lived with this malady life-long see a major decrease in the frequency and severity of their headaches after they reach age 55. Some doctors attribute this decrease to the hardening of the arteries that comes with aging.

For other seniors, though, headaches begin to show up in the golden years. This situation should be a cause for concern and a prompt medical evaluation. Why? Very often, new-onset headaches in older people are symptomatic of a medical condition that needs to be diagnosed and treated.

Basically, the senior migraine picture boils down to this: Because older folks are subject to a wider realm of health problems just by virtue of having bodies that are older, they need to report to their doctors any new or oddball headaches. The head pain may simply be a migraine of old age, or it may be more serious — a sign of a health condition that urgently needs evaluation and treatment (see Chapter 23). Either way, a senior needs a doctor's evaluation for help with pain relief.

Losing Migraine Pain along with Your Hair

While you may dislike some aspects of growing older (thinning hair, expanding waist, arthritis pains), you're sure to love and appreciate the gradual fading away of your migraines. After years of battling them and having them invade your plans, family, and workplace, your headaches seem to go on sabbatical — and your hope is that they never return.

The migraineur who experiences a decrease in the severity and frequency of headaches in her early 50s will usually notice this reversal of ill fortune just get better and better. You may be in disbelief at first — truly, the change seems too good to be true — but your doctor probably told you that you had this phase to look forward to. Here it is, a break at last from regular bouts of migraine pain, nausea, and other symptoms.

No one really seems to know why migraines become less severe and more infrequent as we age. But many migraineurs report far less trouble with headaches after they pass the age of 50. (For other types of headaches, this reduced frequency may not be the case.)

After your migraines go away, a splitting headache is cause for concern. So if you haven't had bad head pain for years, and a headache pops up one day, see a doctor as soon as possible, because it may well be a sign of a serious health condition.

Gaining Wisdom and Migraines

One of the strangest aspects of migraines is their individualistic nature, which makes them difficult to understand and rather hard to treat. For some people who pass the 50 mark, migraines are part and parcel of their senior years. In rare cases, they show up for the first time ever, baffling the brand-new migraine sufferer. Why now?

About a third of the time, migraines in the senior years are caused by a medical condition. Although you may automatically think "yikes, brain tumor!" it's much more likely that your migraines are the result of a medication you're taking, glaucoma, high blood pressure, arthritis, or a sleep problem. But because you can't know for sure what's going on, it's important to have a medical evaluation.

Often, in older folks, headaches aren't serious — they may be tension-type, cluster, or migraine headaches.

Folks older than 50 who have been fairly headache-free are more likely than younger ones to have a serious or life-threatening cause behind their headache — including glaucoma, kidney disease, tumor, stroke, or high blood pressure. Therefore, it's important to see a doctor if you're having headaches for the first time after age 50. Your doctor can determine whether you need tests (see Chapter 6) or just a prescription for a pain reliever.

Some medications commonly used by seniors, such as some high blood pressure drugs and medications taken for angina, can be headache-makers.

Don't try to improvise treatment by taking a migraine medication used by a friend or your mate. The pill you borrow may not interact well with a health condition you have or other drugs you take regularly. This bad interaction may result in a complication or mask the signs of a serious illness.

Adjusting lifestyle headache triggers

Assuming that other headache causes have been ruled out and you've been diagnosed with migraines, you — a 50-plus migraineur — may need to make lifestyle changes in regard to things that appear to be triggering your headaches. (Chapters 3, 11, and 13 walk you through finding and managing migraine triggers.)

One thing about migraines that many experts agree on is the idea that they can be egged on by up-and-down blips on your brain's radar screen. In other words, the more consistency you have as far as sleep habits, movement, and environmental input, the less likely your triggers will unite and cause you grief in the form of a headache.

Regular exercise, a good diet, and ample rest are all simple adjuncts to your main migraine-fighting plan.

Don't underestimate the importance of making simple changes. The more you can do to streamline your lifestyle and make things less bumpy for your brain, the better your chances of subduing your migraines.

Making dietary changes as needed

If you're new to the migraine headache realm, you may have no idea what types of food or drink are your own personal headache triggers.

It won't take long for you to discover that monitoring what you eat can be a cumbersome undertaking, but keeping a food diary is one of the best ways to get on top of your triggers. (See the headache journal in Chapter 3, and check out Chapter 11 for advice on finding and ridding yourself of headache-prompting food and drink.)

Seeing Your Doctor for Help

Don't try to go it alone. If you're new to headaches — or you've had them for years but never coped especially well — get a healthcare provider on board to help you work up a migraine management plan (see Chapter 5).

Perhaps the treatment you used in the past for pain relief is no longer working. If so, you need to reassess your situation and have your doctor evaluate you.

Investigating health conditions that cause headaches

Have your doctor examine you to rule out the possibility that your brand-new headaches may be indications of an altered health situation.

It used to be that doctors automatically diagnosed depression when a senior complained of headaches. Today, healthcare providers believe that newly occurring headaches in people older than 50 probably don't have a psychological origin.

Some health conditions may cause seniors to develop headaches. These types of headaches include the following:

- **Cervical spondylosis headache:** A dull back-of-the-head headache that gets worse when you move your neck often accompanies cervical disk disease. In older people, changes of cervical spondylosis (or degenerative arthritis in the neck), which aren't unusual, are frequently seen on x-ray films of the neck.

  This pain can be treated with medications such as acetaminophen (Tylenol) or celecoxib (Celebrex), but the treatment varies depending on the individual's other medical conditions.

- **The headache of a transient ischemic attack:** This headache is often nondescript, dull, and moderate. It may last from minutes to hours. The headache itself may act as a precursor of other *brain ischemia symptoms* (symptoms that result from inadequate blood flow), such as weakness on one side of the body or slurred speech.

  Although a transient ischemic attack is similar to a stroke, its effects aren't permanent — they resolve within 24 hours. Along with a headache, you may experience dizziness, weakness in your arm and/or leg on one side of your body, confusion, visual disturbances, coordina-tion problems, and/or slurred speech.

The cause of a transient ischemic attack is a brief interruption in blood flow to the brain from a blood clot or an artery that is narrowed due to *arteriosclerosis* (hardening of the arteries). Your doctor will treat you with an anticoagulant, aspirin, or ticlopidine, with the goal being preven-tion of a full-blown stroke. To keep the attacks from happening again, it's important to make some lifestyle alterations, such as quitting smoking. In some cases, surgery is necessary to correct the narrowed artery.

✔ **Hunger headaches:** Seniors may fail to eat enough food for several dif-ferent reasons. They may be less active due to decreased mobility, and their taste buds may have dulled the pleasure of eating. So they go to a nearby cafeteria at 4:30 in the afternoon for an early dinner, chow down on a senior special, and that's it. They're full. Or so they think.

Another possibility may be that the senior doesn't have adequate access to food — maybe she consumes toast and coffee until her daughter stops by with her daily meal. Obviously, this situation would need to be addressed.

Skipping a meal or not eating enough can result in a drop in blood sugar. The treatment is simple — you need to fuel up regularly. Try to graze, eating five or six small meals spaced out during the day. Make sure that you get ample nutrients, including protein and complex carbohydrates.

✔ **Hypnic headache:** This rare headache (seen most often in people 65 and older) is known for head pain that's bad enough to wake you up at night. The hypnic headache is felt on both sides of the head, is often accompa-nied by nausea, and occurs almost every day during sleep or daytime naps. You may have this sleep-related benign headache several nights per week in the early-morning hours. The headache usually lasts two hours or less. Its cause is unknown.

To prevent more hypnic headache episodes from occurring, doctors treat the headache sufferer with lithium. If you can't tolerate the side effects of lithium (trembling, impaired memory), you can try taking caf-feine in a tablet or drink before you go to bed at night.

✔ **Intracranial tumors or hematomas:** Brain tumors and *chronic subdural hematomas* (a collection of blood on the brain) are more common in the elderly. The headaches caused by intracranial masses aren't always accompanied by nausea or other symptoms, contrary to popular belief.

Some symptoms associated with a brain tumor are the following:

- A dull headache of moderate intensity with no throbbing
- Head pain gets worse with movement
- The headache comes on slowly and progresses, but it can also come and go

- Nausea and vomiting

- You wake up with a headache and find that it gets worse after you get out of bed

Chronic subdural hematomas aren't unusual in older people because of the increased problem of poor balance, which can lead to falls (and thus, head trauma). If you have signs of a hematoma or lesion, your doctor will probably do a CT scan or MRI (see Chapter 6 for more info on these tests) in order to diagnose the problem. If he finds a tumor or hematoma, the situation will probably require surgery. Signs of a sub-dural hematoma include headache, drowsiness, confusion, and (rarely) one-sided weakness.

✔ **Temporal arteritis:** This rare and very serious condition, which is also called giant cell arteritis, is found mostly in elderly people and is associated with new-onset headaches. The headache is usually felt as a continuous throbbing pain in the temples, and the pain gets worse over time until it's with you constantly. Usually, the headache pain is felt on both sides of the head. You may have shoulder and pelvic-area joint or muscle aches and stiffness. You may feel ill and tired, and have tenderness in the temple area over the affected artery. Early diagnosis is important so that treatment can be started promptly to prevent blindness.

Most people who suffer from temporal arteritis must take steroids for months. Unfortunately, there can be multiple side effects with long-term steroid use, including weight gain and an increased risk of osteoporosis. But if temporal arteritis goes untreated, blindness is a definite possibility.

In rare cases, a headache may be a sign of a tumor, aneurysm, or subdural hematoma (a collection of blood on the brain). An *aneurysm* is a balloonlike bulge in the wall of a blood vessel that may rupture or leak blood slowly, causing an awful headache that's sometimes accompanied by vomiting and a stiff neck. With a tumor, the head pain gets worse over time and is sometimes accompanied by *projectile vomiting* (when you vomit, the substance flies from your mouth like a spewing fountain), visual problems, trouble with balance or coordination, and personality and speech changes. A subdural hematoma is often caused by head trauma, but it may sometimes result from a ruptured aneurysm.

If you're 55 or older, your risk of stroke is greater than it was when you were younger. Headaches are common in about a fourth of stroke cases.

A headache associated with stroke can cause pain anywhere on your head. You may vomit, feel dizzy, disoriented, or weak, and experience visual disturbances, paralysis, slurred speech, or difficulty with coordination. You may also breathe irregularly, have a seizure, go into a coma, or die. The stroke occurs as a result of a blocked blood vessel, a blood vessel that is bleeding in the brain, or a blood clot that travels to the brain and blocks an artery.

If in doubt, check it out

A retired teacher saw a health expert on television talking about serious health problems that can cause migraines in people older than 55. The television show put her on a roller coaster of worry about her health. She had always had migraine headaches, but lately she started having a brand-new type of headache that she found a little alarming. On one side of her head at the temple, she had a piercing pain that would come and go. This headache pain had been going on for five days. It wasn't the usual awful migraine pain, but the odd nature of it worried this woman.

She had put off going to the doctor just to save the money. Because she was a 60-year-old retired woman living on a small fixed income, every penny counted. But finally, she was agonizing many hours a day about the possibility of having temporal arteritis — and it was interfering with her daytime TV soaps — so she made an appointment to see her internist.

He examined her and saw no signs of temporal arteritis. He then ran a diagnostic blood test to determine whether he was looking at temporal arteritis. The doctor told her that he didn't think she had the condition, but he was administering the test to put her mind at ease. He also told her that temporal arteritis is a rare condition, and in patients he had seen, the headache was felt on both sides (bilateral) of the head. He felt she was describing head pain that wasn't actually a headache but a result of her grinding her teeth during sleep.

The blood test showed just what the doctor expected. He told his patient to take Aleve whenever the situation comes up again. He told her that if she continued to have this particular kind of pain, she could get a mouthpiece (from her dentist) that would keep her from grinding down her teeth.

As it turned out, going to the doctor provided peace of mind. It was definitely worth the $20 co-payment she had to fork out.

If you think that you may be having a stroke, get immediate medical attention. Call 911, or have someone take you to the ER.

Getting a prescription drug that works with your other meds

If you're a senior (or even if you're younger), warding off the possibility of adverse drug interactions is a prime consideration when your healthcare provider is treating your headaches.

After your doctor determines that your recurring headaches are "just" headaches and not indicative of a more life-threatening condition, you'll need a form of medication that you can use occasionally and that will jibe with other drugs that you take on a regular basis.

Many seniors take some type of prescription medication, so being vigilant for drug interactions is an important part of choosing a migraine painkiller. When you're using a drug for migraines, be sure to report to your doctor any side effects that occur that are disconcerting or aren't among the ones your doctor (or the prescription information sheet) lists.

Many of the drugs often taken by people 50 and older can cause headaches. Some examples are cardiovascular drugs, respiratory system drugs, and central nervous system drugs.

Looking Out for Eye Problems and Atypical Head Pain

If you experience headaches associated with eye problems after age 50, you definitely need to report them to your healthcare provider, because the combination of symptoms will arouse your doctor's suspicions that specific problems may be causing your headaches. Another problem that should be checked out by your doctor is unfamiliar and sudden lancelike facial pain, which can point to trigeminal neuralgia (see "Reporting pain in your face," later in this chapter).

Eye problems associated with headaches may be a sign of developed glaucoma (which requires prompt treatment) or another medical condition. As we discuss earlier in this chapter, temporal arteritis is another condition that can result in headaches and vision loss. No one needs to remind you, of course, that you want to save your vision.

Noting any throbbing pain behind your eyes

If you have a throbbing pain behind one or both eyes, or in your forehead, it may point to glaucoma. The visual symptoms that are sometimes reported with glaucoma include a cloudy film creeping over the eyeball, blurred vision, blind spots, and reduced peripheral vision. Nausea is also a common symptom.

The reason that glaucoma develops in the first place is usually because impaired drainage leads to a fluid buildup in the eye, which spins off into increased pressure inside the eye.

Biting the bullet and getting help

A woman we know has been dealing with her headaches on her own for most of her life. At 73, she lost her sister to cancer and had to live alone, which made her suffering even worse and more isolating when she got a migraine. People believed her when she said, "oh, I'll be fine," even though she really wasn't.

Then she read an article that encouraged migraine sufferers to establish some kind of control over their situation. The article referred to "pain behind the eye" headaches that could be indicative of glaucoma; this really frightened her.

She went to see her healthcare provider at a clinic in Carmel, California, where she lives. The doctor linked her to a support group so that she would have people to talk to — and he encouraged her to make a few lifestyle changes to tone down her headache triggers. (For years, she suspected that the MSG, or monosodium glutamate, in Chinese food led to her headaches, yet she still kept eating it; she seemed to forget between headaches.) The doctor gave her a prescription medication that staved off most of her migraines. She also saw an eye doctor and was told that her eye pressure was normal — no evidence of glaucoma!

"Why didn't I do this years ago?" she wondered, thinking of all the time she had lost suffering with headaches. The bottom line, though, was that she finally felt in charge of her health, and that made living alone much less daunting. When a migraine hit, she took her prescription drug and went to bed to sleep it off. When she woke up, she could call a member of her support group just to touch base and talk about what she went through. The human element proved to be a key part of improving her quality of life considerably.

Angle-closure glaucoma (whose symptoms are redness and pain in or around one eye, a bad headache, blurred vision, and nausea/vomiting) is an emergency. If you experience the symptoms of angle-closure glaucoma, you need to see an eye doctor (ophthalmologist) as soon as possible, because vision can be permanently lost within 48 to 72 hours.

Open-angle glaucoma is a much more common condition. It results in the loss of peripheral vision over a period of many years. If this condition is diagnosed by a yearly eye exam, medications can be prescribed to help control the progression of vision loss.

Most at risk for glaucoma are African-Americans and Asians; people with nearsightedness, an eye injury in their past, or a family history of glaucoma, diabetes, or high blood pressure; and people who have a history of steroid use.

People who are older than 40 and are at increased risk for glaucoma, and all people older than 60, should have yearly eye exams and measurements of the pressure within the eyes.

If you have symptoms of glaucoma, seek treatment immediately. Vision loss can result if you wait too long. The right medications or laser surgery can prevent further vision loss and help your headaches at the same time.

Reporting pain in your face

Trigeminal neuralgia (also called tic douloureux) causes an unbearable facial pain that feels like jabbing or burning and may be described as "shooting." The pain may start near one side of your mouth and then shoot toward your ear, or it may be felt around your ear when you chew; it usually lasts for only a few seconds. A blast of cold air may also cause this facial pain.

Trigeminal neuralgia is a rare disease that's seen more often in women than men. It's also more common in people who are middle-aged or older.

This condition typically responds well to medication. But if the medication fails to work, surgery may be necessary.

In rare cases, trigeminal neuralgia can be a sign of an underlying problem such as multiple sclerosis or a brain tumor, especially in younger patients.

Part VII
The Part of Tens

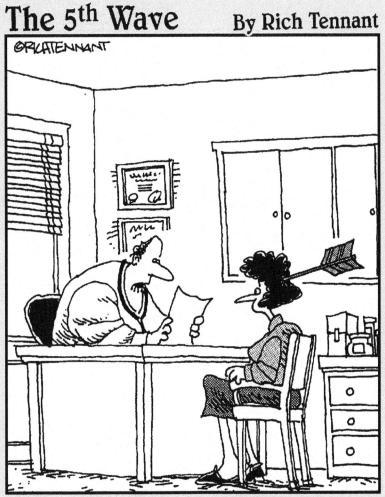

The 5th Wave   By Rich Tennant

"Well, according to our tests, your headaches aren't migraines after all."

In this part . . .

This part covers a few issues that affect migraine folks but defy being classified in any of the other six parts. You get ten tips for dealing effectively with migraine-free folks. Then, for the relative/supporter/friend who wants to be there for a migraine sufferer, we offer ten things you can do to really, truly help. And finally, we tell you eleven ways *not* to treat a migraine — these things just make matters worse (*ouch!*).

Chapter 24

Ten Tips for Dealing with Folks Who Don't Get Migraines

*B*rown eyes, blue eyes. Slim build, athletically inclined. Strong teeth, cavity-prone. When people were diving into the gene pool for traits, maybe you accidentally got in the line for migraine headaches when you thought you were signing up for patience and an even temperament.

Well let's hope that you walked away from the gene lottery with both of those traits, too, because they definitely come in handy when you're dealing with all the folks who don't get or don't understand migraines.

Migraines are troublesome enough, but headache-free folks who start babbling feel-better tips or making their skepticism all too clear — "How could migraines really hurt all that much?" — can give you a real headache.

In response to being misunderstood, your emotions may run the gamut from frustration to embarrassment to anger. But, in the final analysis, you'll just get irritated at yourself if you engage in justification or self-defense. A better plan is to hone a steadfast unwillingness to tell others when your head is hurting and avoid comments and advice from folks who are unsympathetic and suspicious.

You can always take the high road. The following tips can help you deal with the headache-free of this world — and make the encounters time-worthy and energy-worthy.

Express Your Envy (At Least to Yourself)

Give yourself permission to be a teensy-weensy bit envious. Sure, you wish you didn't have migraines. But the person you're envying probably wishes he didn't have buck teeth, depression, or poor vision.

Still, it's okay to admit that you feel the green-eyed monster when you're hit with a headache that keeps you from doing things you like to do. Go ahead and acknowledge your feeling, and then get on with your life.

Shrug Off Unhelpful Advice

Naturally, you may run across people who think that you're embellishing on your headache pain. They may want to help you with a cheery piece of advice about getting over it: "Buck up and you'll feel a whole lot better."

For some reason, this advice can feel almost as bad as a bodybuilder giving you advice on abdominal crunches the first time you visit a gym. Somehow you know he'll be partying with hot chicks way before you polish off washboard abs. And, by the same token, it will be a chilly day in Demonville before a headache-free person manages to eradicate your migraines via positive thinking. Say nothing in response. They probably mean well.

Let others' misunderstandings of you make you a more tolerant person: You can really stretch yourself by remembering that absolutely everyone has a story behind what he does, so don't be too quick to criticize.

Keep a Sense of Perspective

When someone gives you the "I feel so sorry for you" stuff to a nauseating degree, come back with a "Hey, I'm really not that bad off, and soon I'll be feeling great again!"

Enlighten that person by letting him know that having migraines doesn't mean you're incapacitated or handicapped. You're mostly just inconvenienced. Don't react with shame or frustration — show your jaunty attitude.

Steel Yourself for the Very Irritating

Some friends or relatives may be especially irksome with the things they say or the way they act around you in regard to your headaches. So brace yourself when you know you'll be around someone who's bothersome — and get ready to be extra patient.

Chances are, these annoying people have a way of irking pretty much everyone around them, so it's not like you're being singled out for abuse.

Try to Love Even the Headache-Free

You're the only one of five kids who inherited your mother's migraines. It's unfortunate, yes, but that's no reason to get mad at your siblings. Remember, your siblings didn't get a 100-percent perfect package of genetics either, so try to dilute your desire to make them responsible for not having the headache gene.

Be Matter-of-Fact about Having to Miss Engagements

If you have to miss a special occasion because you're sick with a migraine, state the truth, and don't feel bad about it. Immunize yourself to the nagging you hear, and do what you think is best for your health.

Warn People Up Front

Let's say that you sign up to help at a food pantry. Your heart is in the right place, and you hope to be there every single week. But you're afraid that you may not win any perfect-attendance awards, because a migraine may force you to cancel occasionally.

You can lessen your stress by simply letting the pantry director know up front: "I have migraines occasionally, but I'll be as consistent in my volunteer work as I possibly can. And I'll call if I can't come." Telling the director about your situation will make you feel better, and it will help other folks with their planning (and their understanding of you as a person).

Don't Let Anyone Guilt-Trip You

Backing out of social obligations and workplace duties may make some affected person want to put you in your place: "Well, you really let us down."

Or, "I wish you'd told us days ago that you weren't coming to my son's bar mitzvah — I had a special place reserved for you next to a friend of mine from out of town who wanted to meet you."

The guilt card is one that's especially difficult for migraine sufferers to handle. You probably feel guilty enough before you pick up the phone to call and express your regrets, and having someone add his own assessment to the mix doesn't make things any better.

But there's really not much you can do to improve matters. Grant that person the right to be disappointed, and grant yourself the right to know that you have a good reason for not attending. You know that your migraines improve much faster when you're able to lie down in a dark room after taking your migraine medication.

Plus, you're highly aware that it's impossible for a migraineur to inform some-one in advance that he's going to have a headache! Your migraine rarely e-mails you an estimated time of arrival!

Help Your Hosts Accommodate Your Triggers

Have compassion for the frustrations that others experience on your behalf. You're going to a friend's house for dinner, but your host wants to serve Chinese food — *problem*. Your guest wants to play loud music, but he's heard that loud noises can spur a migraine — *problem*. You've been invited to a wine tasting, but the hostess has no idea what to do with a non-drinker like you — *problem*.

Do what you can to ease your hosts' worries: "Don't fix anything special for me. I'll eat a snack before I come to your dinner and just enjoy everyone's company." Or, "I can move myself out onto the patio where the music won't be a problem for me." Or, "I've been to wine tastings before, and I had fun socializing and listening to everyone taste and talk. I had even more fun lis-tening to great gossip after all those [inebriated] tongues starting wagging."

Express Your Disappointment at Missing Important Events

Be endearing and kind so that people who are disappointed by your non-attendance won't take your absence personally.

You want to go to your daughter's college graduation more than anything. She's an honor graduate, and you're dying to see those gold cords draped around her shoulders and hear her name called out. You're a proud parent, indeed. But you're vomiting, and your head feels like it's splitting in two. Going to graduation in your shape would only be a problem for all concerned, not to mention next to impossible.

So do what you can do under the circumstances: Write a sweet note. Tell your child that you'll be there in spirit and you'd give anything to be able to go.

One woman recalls the deep sadness she felt when her father missed her high school graduation (when she was valedictorian and delivered the commencement address) and college graduation (when she was one of the ten top students). "I'll admit I wanted him there for selfish reasons — I was pretty proud of myself, and desperately wanted him to say he was, too. My mother did come, and my husband and brother, but I desperately missed my dad. I just wish he'd let me know that it mattered to him, too." Many years later, her father told her how distraught he had been at having to miss her graduations, and that, at the time, he didn't know what to say — so he said nothing.

Children and teens are often the most confused when a migraine-suffering parent misses a major event but shows no remorse or disappointment. The kid may walk away with the idea that the headache was an "easy way out," and that the things he does really don't matter very much.

Your job is to provide ample reassurance. Let your children know that you're as disappointed as they are when your migraines make you miss important occasions. Send a "wish I were there" memento or note. When your child gets home, and you're feeling better, ask for details and pictures. If you show your interest and affection, they'll survive their disappointment, knowing full well that you would have loved to have gone.

Many migraineurs rarely miss work or outside activities. You don't automatically have to bail just because you have a headache (see the chapters in Part V). In fact, many migraine sufferers use headache preventives and remedies so handily (see Chapters 7 and 8), that only a rare attack makes them miss an important event.

Chapter 25

Ten Things You Can Do for the Migraine Sufferer You Love

*L*ove those headaches away! That's exactly what you'd like to do for the dearly beloved migraine sufferer in your inner circle, but it isn't something you can do. So you must summon up that fabled "wisdom to know the difference."

In fact, you may feel like a big third-wheel when you're watching someone you love writhing in pain with a migraine headache. From the viewpoint of the headache sufferer, that's really not the case.

Actually, there's a great deal of comfort in knowing that someone cares — that your friend or mate is ready to fetch a cold compress for your head, prepare you a bowl of chicken-noodle soup, or zip into a drive-through for a vanilla shake and a burger.

What's not comforting for a migraineur, however, is the mate, friend, or child who tells them to pull themselves up by the bootstraps, cheer up, or get a grip. This "advice" is *so* not helpful. The last thing a sick person needs to hear is that she will get better if she just tries.

The best way to comfort a migraineur is to just jump in and do what you can (in a low-key and quiet way) to be a source of sustenance and support.

You may feel extremely frustrated and helpless when your mate gets an awful headache. That's natural. Of course, you've probably seen the symptoms before, and you've always hated the way migraines can be so debilitating and cause so much suffering. But it's your job, as one who loves a headache-prone person, to be on standby when a headache strikes, ready to help if needed. You need to maintain a relatively silent vigil. Make no demands, ask no questions, and expect no witty repartee.

The following sections cover ten things you can do for the migraine sufferer you love.

Be On Call

Be ready to fly into action if called. Express your willingness to go to the pharmacy, store, or fast-food eatery. Do what you can to take the load of duties off the person who's suffering.

Stay Cheerful

Keep your attitude upbeat, not somber. But don't try to engage the migraineur in conversation.

Talking is one of the hardest things to do for a person who's sick with a headache. She may want to talk, but it's tough when her mind is in a sling. So be kind, and don't make your friend overexert her brain. If you start a conversation, she'll try to accommodate you (that's what migraine folks do), but she may feel worse if she has to strain her brain — so respect that.

Crank Up Your Compassion

Even if you're not ordinarily a touchy-feely type, this is a great time to learn how to cover up cold extremities, fetch glasses of water, and lower the lights. The little things are often the most welcome and helpful to a person who's experiencing a head-throbbing extravaganza of sensory miseries.

Resist the Urge to Cajole

You may want to urge your loved one to try to get better so that you can go to the party of the year or the company picnic, but don't do it. If you need to go somewhere, go by yourself. Don't press a migraineur to get up and socialize.

A gut feeling lets a headache sufferer know when she can be active and when she can't. Your pressure doesn't help matters. It just makes her feel guilty for being a wet blanket.

Serve as a Social Secretary

Answer the phone, take messages, and make excuses for social engagements. Go to the store, drive the carpool, and stand in at the soccer game.

Remember not to give out personal information about the migraineur or her condition unless she tells you that it's okay.

Take Charge of the Kids

If a migraine sufferer's head is hurting, she'll find it hard to take care of small children. As a friend or mate, you may be able to assist by cajoling the small fry of the house into understanding that mom is temporarily out of commission and needs a bit of quiet.

It is truly too much to ask a person suffering with a migraine to keep her kids quiet (when she's already feeling awful about missing time with them).

Make Necessary Work-Related Phone Calls

Does the migraineur's employer need to be told that your friend or spouse can't come to work today or may be coming in late?

Of course, the best route is for the migraine sufferer to phone her employer herself, but that may be impossible. She may need you to place that important call if she's incapacitated.

Call the Doc if the Headache Worsens

Watch for signs that migraine pain, nausea, and/or vomiting are getting worse. If these symptoms get worse, call your loved one's doctor. Don't try to diagnose the situation — just call for help if there is any sign that alarms you (see Chapter 18).

Be Thoughtful

Put flowers in the room. Close the drapes if the light is bothersome. Ask whether the migraineur wants to listen to some soft music. Do what you can to help the sufferer endure the period of isolation.

Ask What You Can Do

The best question you can ask is "What can I do to help?" If the migraineur finds back-tickling relaxing, and you're up for it, do it. If she enjoys hearing things such as "I hope you feel better soon," say these things. If she wants you and everyone else out of sight, try to make it happen.

Ask any migraine sufferer — it's absolutely wonderful to know that someone is nearby, eager to cater to your needs and fully aware that you're hurting and miserable. Sometimes the mere presence of a mate or friend is enough to make the hurting party feel hopeful that the end of the pain can't be far away. Lying in bed in a tunnel of agony can be a desolate and lonely feeling, especially when migraines aren't isolated incidents.

Because you love this individual, put your own wants and needs on the back burner while you help her recuperate. A true friend knows when to lie low and serve as a loving helpmate.

Chapter 26

Eleven Ways NOT to Treat a Migraine

. . . .

In This Chapter

▷ Showing evidence of your migraine-savvy

▷ Making sure that you stay faithful to your management plan

▷ Sidestepping the trap of thinking that your migraine triggers are no longer triggers

. . . .

*Y*ou know how it is with migraines — there are some things you can do and some things you can't. But one rule should be an out-and-out federal law: Don't repeat mistakes you made in the past. And that's what we mean by "ways NOT to treat a migraine."

To highlight the importance of relying on a valid headache plan (and not zigzagging madly into the land of improvisation), here are 11 very important ways *not* to treat a migraine.

Go Off Your Program

Sure, you know that you get headaches from MSG. Or red wine. Or peanuts. But you still want to believe that your triggers will lose their oomph someday. This probably isn't going to happen. So it's far better to stick to the migraine management plan that you devised — don't go veering off on side streets.

Methodical folks are unlikely to have trouble with migraine pain after they get their management plan worked out. But the wafflers of this world, the people who experience a brand-new world almost every day, are often too quick to abandon or forget the basics — and oops, their headache does it again.

So try to be sensible and practical. You can't rewrite your migraine-attack plan each time the weather changes. Do what works, and stick to it.

If you pick up some new tips along the way, you can incorporate them into your migraine-attack plan. But don't go changing too much after you discover what works for keeping your headaches in line. If your migraine-relieving strategies have accomplished the goals of reduced frequency and severity, why not adhere to them?

Take Too Many Drugs

One day, you throw caution to the wind and take someone else's drugs. Another day, you experiment with several different medications during the several hours that you're fighting a migraine.

Don't do it! Experimenting with drugs that aren't on your headache management plan may result in nasty drug interactions and perhaps even a horrible migraine. You need to run your ideas past your doctor and get an okay first.

Ignore Dosage Recommendations

You received some sound advice from a healthcare provider about how much of a certain pain-relief medication you should take — and how often. So, don't start improvising: "Oh, that helped a little bit, so I'll take twice as much an hour from now."

Don't do it! Knowing how much of your medication to take, and when to take that amount, is a critical part of getting good results. If you go jogging off the path of good medicine, you may end up with worse problems than a bad headache.

Believe Crazy Claims

"If you'll just put your head in the vise and let me drill a few holes, you'll never have migraines again." Off-the-wall treatments may sound intriguing, but be sure to run past your doctor anything that you want to add to your headache treatment plan. Unless you have a medical background, you probably aren't qualified to weed through bogus product claims and pinpoint alternatives that are actually legitimate.

Sure, plenty of hucksters may want to sell you a crystal ball for predicting when a headache is coming, or a magic carpet that will zap migraine energy when you start feeling bad. But the truth is, you're going to find far more comfort in the kinds of treatments that have been validated for their helpfulness and safety in reducing the pain, nausea, and other symptoms of migraines. Let wacky witch doctors sell their bills of goods to someone else — you're not buying. It's best to keep your head intact — especially for all those days when you don't have a headache and your brain comes in handy.

Keep Taking a Drug that Doesn't Work

Don't keep taking a medication that isn't working or has never worked for you — it probably never will work. Nothing miraculous is going to happen just by virtue of your commitment to a certain drug. Instead, look for a replacement. Get with your doctor and try a different direction.

Try to Gut it Out and Go Out

When you're feeling very sick and incapacitated, you may try to keep a stiff upper lip, gut it out, and go someplace.

Of course, you don't want to miss anything, and that's a real motivator. But going places when you're way too sick is always a mistake. Chances are, you won't make it through the activity, and you'll be forced to cut the fun short and drive yourself home. Or you may wind up too sick to drive, and then you'll be in a real fix.

Stuff Yourself with Tons of Food

Migraineurs have been known to overeat, thinking that it may knock down their pain a few notches. They've tried everything else, for heaven's sake!

But food-stuffing won't do any good. The only reason your headache may seem to disappear right after you eat is probably just lucky timing — your headache is already on the wane. As a side note, packing on extra pounds probably isn't going to make you happy, either.

Try the Sun-and-Activity Remedy

Someone may try to convince you that you'll feel better if you just get out of bed and go to a festival or county fair. "A little sunshine, a beer or two, and a turkey leg, and you'll be as good as new."

Not so fast there. It isn't very likely that sun and full-tilt activity (or alcohol) will make you feel better if you're already in the throes of a bad migraine. In fact, these activities are likely to aggravate migraines.

On the other hand, if you have nothing more than the nagging edge of a headache, you may want to take some medication and go ahead with your plans.

Doctor-Hop

You don't like what you hear from one doctor, so you go to another, and another. Soon, you're making a hobby of it.

Seeing one doctor who focuses on your headaches and helps you find answers is a far better use of your time and money. When you find a medical advisor who understands you and can help you manage your migraines, stick with him. Pay attention to his suggestions until, together, you devise a headache management plan that works for you.

Foster a Sick-Person Reputation

A gut feeling tells you that, despite what your doctor says, you really won't get well. You fear that you'll face debilitating migraines forever. Nothing is going to work for you.

One good way to make sure that you'll always have headaches is to get real comfy with the victim role — decide that all the coddling and TLC is pretty nice. If you take this approach, you'll only help give migraine sufferers a bad name.

Become an ER Junkie

For you, it's too much trouble to see a specialist and set up a migraine management plan. Instead, you just head for the emergency room when you get a bad headache.

Bad plan. People who are frequent flyers in the ER have several big problems. The staff may begin to dismiss your complaints because you cry wolf too often. Furthermore, you may build up a tolerance to the medications you're given time after time. And, you may also become a drug-abuse suspect.

Take the time to see a headache specialist and find out the real scoop on what you should be doing — instead of just flying by the seat of your pants every time you have a migraine attack.

Index

• E •

• *Q* •

• *R* •

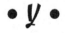

NOW AVAILABLE!

FOR DUMMIES Videos & DVDs

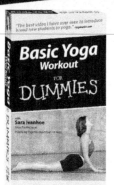

Basic Yoga Workout FOR DUMMIES
with Sara Ivanhoe

An Easy-to-Follow Yoga Practice

Instructor Sara Ivanhoe offers step-by-step instruction of the 12 essential yoga postures. This workout shows you proper technique, as well as tips on modifying postures for your fitness level. Today, many people use yoga to help alleviate back pain, reduce stress, and increase flexibility.

VHS - 45 Mins. $9.99
DVD - 70 Mins. $14.98

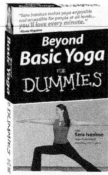

Beyond Basic Yoga FOR DUMMIES
with Sara Ivanhoe

An Easy-to-Follow Workout

The *Beyond Basic Yoga Workout For Dummies* is the next step for anyone who has enjoyed *Basic Yoga Workout For Dummies* and is ready to enhance their practice with 12 more postures. This workout is a little more advanced than the basic yoga program but still features the *For Dummies* format.

VHS - 45 Mins. $9.99
DVD - 55 Mins. $14.98

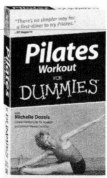

Pilates Workout FOR DUMMIES
with Michelle Dozois

An Easy-to-Follow Workout

Instructor Michelle Dozois offers step-by-step instruction of 18 popular Pilates mat exercises to help you strengthen and lengthen your muscles, improve your posture, and tone and tighten your midsection.

VHS - 40 Mins. $9.99
DVD - 60 Mins. $14.98

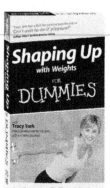

Shaping Up with Weights FOR DUMMIES
with Tracy York

An Easy-to-Follow Workout

Instructor Tracy York offers step-by-step instruction of 12 key strength-training exercises and makes it easy to work out at any level. This workout incorporates both upper- and lower-body exercises to help tone muscles and burn more calories per day, which leads to fat loss.

VHS - 51 Mins. $9.99

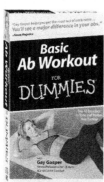

Basic Ab Workout FOR DUMMIES
with Gay Gasper

An Easy-to-Follow Workout

Instructor Gay Gasper demonstrates her top 10 exercises to tone and flatten your tummy. Throughout this workout, she gives you more advanced options for the exercises so you can start at any level and then advance as you become more fit.

VHS - 45 Mins. $9.99
DVD - 55 Mins. $14.98

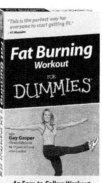

Fat Burning Workout FOR DUMMIES
with Gay Gasper

An Easy-to-Follow Workout

In this workout, instructor Gay Gasper offers step-by-step instructions of the 10 basic exercises that make up any aerobic routine. She incorporates both high- and low-impact choices in an effective workout to help you burn more fat, use more calories every day, and meet your fitness goals.

VHS - 45 Mins. $9.99

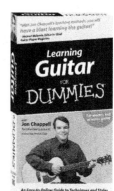

Learning Guitar FOR DUMMIES
with Jon Chappell

An Easy-to-Follow Guide to Techniques and Styles

Instructor Jon Chappell provides step-by-step instruction of all of the skills you need to become an accomplished guitar player! By simply watching the instructor onscreen and following along, you can learn to play songs — without reading music.

VHS - 75 Mins. $12.98
DVD - 75 Mins. $16.98

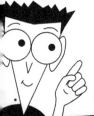

FOR DUMMIES®

The easy way to get more done and have more fun

...NAL FINANCE & BUSINESS

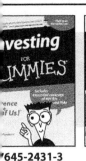

Home Buying

0-7645-2431-3

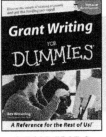

0-7645-5331-3

Grant Writing

0-7645-5307-0

Also available:

Accounting For Dummies
(0-7645-5314-3)

Business Plans Kit For
Dummies
(0-7645-5365-8)

Managing For Dummies
(1-5688-4858-7)

Mutual Funds For Dummies
(0-7645-5329-1)

QuickBooks All-in-One Desk
Reference For Dummies
(0-7645-1963-8)

Resumes For Dummies
(0-7645-5471-9)

Small Business Kit For
Dummies
(0-7645-5093-4)

Starting an eBay Business
For Dummies
(0-7645-1547-0)

Taxes For Dummies 2003
(0-7645-5475-1)

..., GARDEN, FOOD & WINE

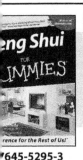

0-7645-5295-3

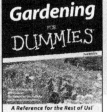

Gardening

0-7645-5130-2

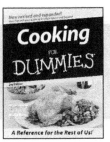

Cooking

0-7645-5250-3

Also available:

Bartending For Dummies
(0-7645-5051-9)

Christmas Cooking For
Dummies
(0-7645-5407-7)

Cookies For Dummies
(0-7645-5390-9)

Diabetes Cookbook For
Dummies
(0-7645-5230-9)

Grilling For Dummies
(0-7645-5076-4)

Home Maintenance For
Dummies
(0-7645-5215-5)

Slow Cookers For Dummies
(0-7645-5240-6)

Wine For Dummies
(0-7645-5114-0)

...SS, SPORTS, HOBBIES & PETS

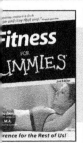

Fitness

0-7645-5167-1

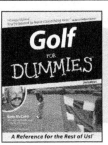

Golf

0-7645-5146-9

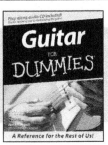

Guitar

0-7645-5106-X

Also available:

Cats For Dummies
(0-7645-5275-9)

Chess For Dummies
(0-7645-5003-9)

Dog Training For Dummies
(0-7645-5286-4)

Labrador Retrievers For
Dummies
(0-7645-5281-3)

Martial Arts For Dummies
(0-7645-5358-5)

Piano For Dummies
(0-7645-5105-1)

Pilates For Dummies
(0-7645-5397-6)

Power Yoga For Dummies
(0-7645-5342-9)

Puppies For Dummies
(0-7645-5255-4)

Quilting For Dummies
(0-7645-5118-3)

Rock Guitar For Dummies
(0-7645-5356-9)

Weight Training For Dummies
(0-7645-5168-X)

...ble wherever books are sold.
www.dummies.com or call 1-877-762-2974 to order direct

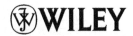

WILEY

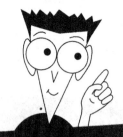

FOR DUMMIES

A world of resources to help you grow

TRAVEL

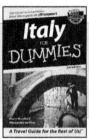

0-7645-5453-0

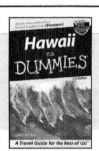

0-7645-5438-7

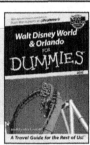

0-7645-5444-1

EDUCATION & TEST PREPARATION

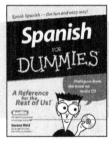

0-7645-5194-9

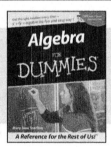

0-7645-5325-9

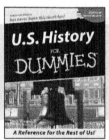

0-7645-5249-X

HEALTH, SELF-HELP & SPIRITUALITY

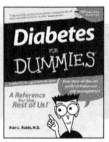

0-7645-5154-X

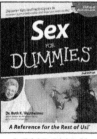

0-7645-5302-X

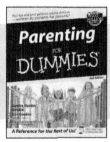

0-7645-5418-2

FOR DUMMIES®

Plain-English solutions for everyday challenges

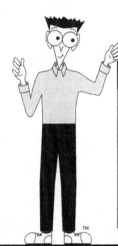

E & BUSINESS COMPUTER BASICS

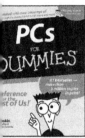 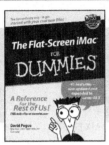 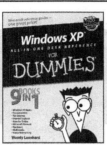

0-7645-0838-5   0-7645-1663-9   0-7645-1548-9

Also available:

Excel 2002 All-in-One Desk Reference For Dummies (0-7645-1794-5)

Office XP 9-in-1 Desk Reference For Dummies (0-7645-0819-9)

PCs All-in-One Desk Reference For Dummies (0-7645-0791-5)

Troubleshooting Your PC For Dummies (0-7645-1669-8)

Upgrading & Fixing PCs For Dummies (0-7645-1665-5)

Windows XP For Dummies (0-7645-0893-8)

Windows XP For Dummies Quick Reference (0-7645-0897-0)

Word 2002 For Dummies (0-7645-0839-3)

RNET & DIGITAL MEDIA

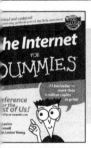 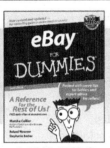 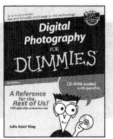

0-7645-0894-6   0-7645-1642-6   0-7645-1664-7

Also available:

CD and DVD Recording For Dummies (0-7645-1627-2)

Digital Photography All-in-One Desk Reference For Dummies (0-7645-1800-3)

eBay For Dummies (0-7645-1642-6)

Genealogy Online For Dummies (0-7645-0807-5)

Internet All-in-One Desk Reference For Dummies (0-7645-1659-0)

Internet For Dummies Quick Reference (0-7645-1645-0)

Internet Privacy For Dummies (0-7645-0846-6)

Paint Shop Pro For Dummies (0-7645-2440-2)

Photo Retouching & Restoration For Dummies (0-7645-1662-0)

Photoshop Elements For Dummies (0-7645-1675-2)

Scanners For Dummies (0-7645-0783-4)

Get smart! Visit www.dummies.com

• **Find listings of even more Dummies titles**

• **Browse online articles, excerpts, and how-to's**

• **Sign up for daily or weekly e-mail tips**

• **Check out Dummies fitness videos and other products**

• **Order from our online bookstore**

Available wherever books are sold. Go to www.dummies.com or call 1-877-762-2974 to order direct

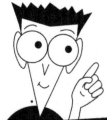

FOR DUMMIES®

Helping you expand your horizons and realize your potent

GRAPHICS & WEB SITE DEVELOPMENT

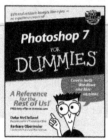

0-7645-1651-5

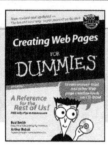

0-7645-1643-4

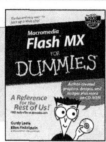

0-7645-0895-4

Also available:

Adobe Acrobat 5 PDF
For Dummies
(0-7645-1652-3)
ASP.NET For Dummies
(0-7645-0866-0)
ColdFusion MX for Dummies
(0-7645-1672-8)
Dreamweaver MX For
Dummies
(0-7645-1630-2)
FrontPage 2002 For Dummies
(0-7645-0821-0)

HTML 4 For Dummies
(0-7645-0723-0)
Illustrator 10 For Dum
(0-7645-3636-2)
PowerPoint 2002 For
Dummies
(0-7645-0817-2)
Web Design For Dumm
(0-7645-0823-7)

PROGRAMMING & DATABASES

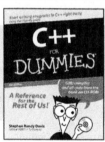

0-7645-0746-X

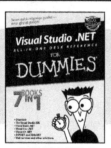

0-7645-1626-4

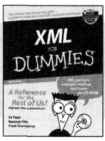

0-7645-1657-4

Also available:

Access 2002 For Dummies
(0-7645-0818-0)
Beginning Programming
For Dummies
(0-7645-0835-0)
Crystal Reports 9 For
Dummies
(0-7645-1641-8)
Java & XML For Dummies
(0-7645-1658-2)
Java 2 For Dummies
(0-7645-0765-6)

JavaScript For Dummi
(0-7645-0633-1)
Oracle9i For Dummies
(0-7645-0880-6)
Perl For Dummies
(0-7645-0776-1)
PHP and MySQL For
Dummies
(0-7645-1650-7)
SQL For Dummies
(0-7645-0737-0)
Visual Basic .NET For
Dummies
(0-7645-0867-9)

LINUX, NETWORKING & CERTIFICATION

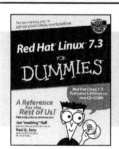

0-7645-1545-4

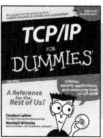

0-7645-1760-0

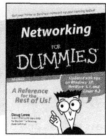

0-7645-0772-9

Also available:

A+ Certification For Dummies
(0-7645-0812-1)
CCNP All-in-One Certification
For Dummies
(0-7645-1648-5)
Cisco Networking For
Dummies
(0-7645-1668-X)
CISSP For Dummies
(0-7645-1670-1)
CIW Foundations For
Dummies
(0-7645-1635-3)

Firewalls For Dummie
(0-7645-0884-9)
Home Networking For
Dummies
(0-7645-0857-1)
Red Hat Linux All-in-O
Desk Reference For Du
(0-7645-2442-9)
UNIX For Dummies
(0-7645-0419-3)

Available wherever books are sold.
Go to www.dummies.com or call 1-877-762-2974 to order direct

CPSIA information can be obtained
at www.ICGtesting.com
Printed in the USA
BVOW08s1918090218
507750BV00001B/1/P